Yoga for a Beautiful Face

Lourdes Julian Doplito Çabuk was born in 1950 in the Philippines and graduated from the University of Santo Tomas with a degree in medical technology.

Her deep interest in art, beauty, and spirituality inspired her to change careers, and at the beginning of the 1980s, she took yoga and healing-crystal training with Master "Osho" Bhagwan Shree Rashneesh.

From the 1970s until the 1990s, she owned a flower shop and a boutique and worked as a florist, decorator, and interior designer in New York City and Orlando, Florida. At the same time, she worked in a jewelry store, where she continued to learn about precious and semiprecious stones.

Starting in the 1990s, Lourdes Julian Doplito gained experience with Hatha yoga, Kundalini yoga, Raja and Kriya yoga, under the supervision of Yoga Master Adnan Ananda Siddviho Çabuk. At his suggestion, she studied topics like "Delaying the Aging Process" and "Natural Beauty." This developed into her "Beauty and Face Yoga" program. Since 2000 she has shared her program and knowledge about Hatha and Kriya yoga at the YAASC Siddashram Yoga Center in Nişantaşi, Istanbul, Turkey.

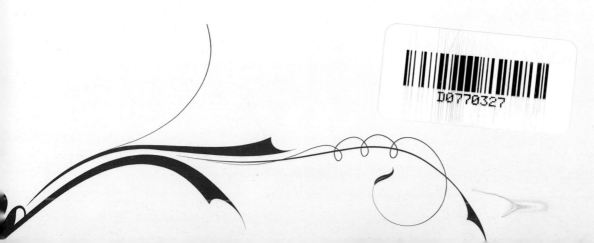

First published 2008 under the title *Güzellik-Gençlik ve Yuz Yogasi*
Text copyright © Lourdes Julian Doplito Çabuk
Book copyright © 2008 Kaknüs Publishing, Istanbul, Turkey
Translation © 2010 Hunter House Inc., Publishers, Alameda, CA

Hunter House Inc., Publishers
PO Box 2914
Alameda CA 94501-0914

Library of Congress Cataloging-in-Publication Data
Çabuk, Lourdes Julian Doplito.
[Gesichts-Yoga. English]
Yoga for a beautiful face : easy exercises to help you look young
again / Lourdes Julian Çabuk. — 1st ed.
    p.   cm.
    ISBN 978-0-89793-526-5 (trade paper)
    1. Hatha yoga—Therapeutic use. 2. Beauty, Personal.
    3. Aging—Prevention—Popular works. I. Title.
RM727.Y64C3313 2009
613.7'046—dc22   2009024811

Ordering
Trade bookstores in the U.S. and Canada please contact:

Publishers Group West
1700 Fourth Street, Berkeley CA 94710
Phone: (800) 788-3123   Fax: (800) 351-5073

Hunter House books are available at bulk discounts for textbook
course adoptions; to qualifying community, health-care, and
government organizations; and for special promotions and
fund-raising. For details please contact:

Special Sales Department
Hunter House Inc., PO Box 2914, Alameda CA 94501-0914
Phone: (510) 865-5282   Fax: (510) 865-4295
E-mail: ordering@hunterhouse.com

Individuals can order our books from most bookstores,
by calling **(800) 266-5592,** or from our website at
www.hunterhouse.com

Printed and bound by Inter Basim Inc., Istanbul, Turkey
Manufactured in Istanbul, Turkey

9 8 7 6 5 4 3 2 1   First U.S. Edition   10 11 12 13 14

Project Credits

Cover Design: Peri Poloni-Gabriel
Book Production: John McKercher
Copywriter: Seda Darcan Çiftçi
Designer: Hatice Dursun
Photographs: Ali Kabaş, Mehmet Acar, Feza Acar
Anatomical Illustrations: Andras Szunyoghy
Translator: Emily Banwell
Copy Editor: Mary Miller
Proofreader: John David Marion
Managing Editor: Alexandra Mummery
Editorial Assistant: Martha Scarpati
Senior Marketing Associate: Reina Santana
Publicity Coordinator: Sean Harvey
Rights Coordinator: Candace Groskreutz
Customer Service Manager: Christina Sverdrup
Order Fulfillment: Washul Lakdhon
Administrator: Theresa Nelson
Computer Support: Peter Eichelberger
Publisher: Kiran S. Rana

Yoga

for a Beautiful Face

EASY EXERCISES TO HELP YOU LOOK YOUNG AGAIN

Lourdes Julian Doplito Çabuk

Translated from the German by Emily Banwell

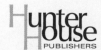

Hunter House
PUBLISHERS

List of Contents

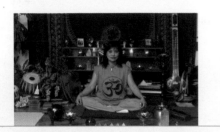

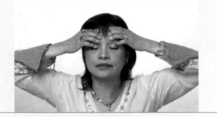

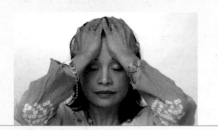

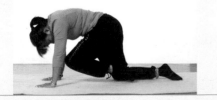

$\mathcal{L}$ist of Contents

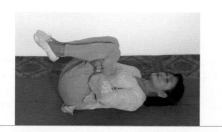

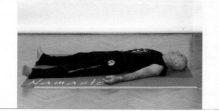

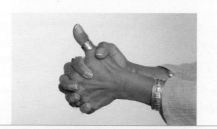

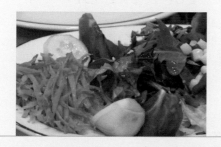

Let our existence be as fragrant as jasmine
pleasant as a breeze in the spring
soft as the flowers in the cotton fields
humble as the water that flows beneath all things
and even stronger than the stones in the riverbed.

Lourdes J. D. Gabuk

Dedication This book is dedicated to my parents, Loretta and Manuel Doplito, who brought me into the world and raised me with a great deal of love. In this same vein, I would like to bow to all mothers and fathers in this world. As they raise their children with much effort and hard work, their only wish is to see those children be happy and successful.

Preface: What Is Yoga?

Many books have already been written about yoga. If you are just beginning yoga, I would recommend choosing just one book to start with. It doesn't matter which book or which type of yoga practice you choose, since in my opinion they all serve the same purpose. The important thing is that you're interested in yoga. You can find many different books and other sources of information, and seek out a variety of yoga teachers, but in the end you will have to do the exercises yourself. Yoga will open a door for you, and the exercises will help guide you along your path to self-fulfillment—that is, your journey of self-discovery.

Don't expect others to give you the energy to find enlightenment! The strength to awaken or increase your inner energy is found in nature. All of the living things surrounding us affect our physical energies. All life forms are made up of molecules, which in turn are made of tiny atoms. Those tiny atoms, the basis of our entire existence, are tied so closely to one another that they can't be seen with the naked eye. Ultimately, our existence rests upon this large network.

Our bodies are always creating new cells, but at the same time, all of our cells are aging and dying off. Our cells are also made of tiny atoms, and the continuous flow of energy enlivens them. Because the human body is always renewing itself and is made up of living cells, the expression "anti-aging" does not correspond to reality. In our day and age, anyway, it is not possible to stop the aging process. Scientists are looking for a magic formula that will allow people to "stay the way they are." Maybe someday we will be able to stop age-related changes in our external appearance, but for now it is more realistic to talk about *delaying* the aging process. Stress is the main factor that causes premature aging. I'm sure you're already conscious of our nonstop daily routines, which are a result of today's technology and the consumption-oriented society in which we live. The stress related to this lifestyle threatens all of us. Some of us are aware of this stress, but others subject themselves to it without realizing what they're doing.

How should we deal with these causes of stress, known or unknown? First, we need to be satisfied with ourselves. We need to create peace within ourselves and start projecting it outward as well. This allows us to face life's challenges with more balance, and that's exactly why I created my "Beauty and Face Yoga" program.

Yoga for a Beautiful Face can help you come to terms with yourself—physically, emotionally, and spiritually. The energy you gain from the program will make it much easier to face life's challenges. Yoga, a style of movement that has been practiced in Asia for thousands of years, can help you grow stronger.

Yoga does not mean a series of acrobatic exercises that need to be done perfectly. Do you know how yoga positions developed? Can you imagine how the yogis, rishis, and sadhus might have developed the yoga practice—a science of the body—thousands of years ago, before people even had books?

Those humble, wise people meditated to find self-fulfillment and become one with the universe; they did so for hours, days, even months. On the path to enlightenment, it was important to live in a healthy body. Their circulation had to keep functioning and their internal organs had to work well. Instinctively, they began to straighten and bend their arms and legs as they meditated, stretching out their bodies or imitating a cat's posture. This was the beginning of the yoga poses.

I would advise everyone who wants to do yoga to first breathe calmly in and out, and then listen to what your body is telling you. Everyone's physical makeup and physical needs are different. It doesn't matter what the yoga exercises you do are called, or how far you can bend or stretch. The important thing is to get to know yourself and to be aware of your physical condition—to be able to evaluate your capabilities and not to overexert yourself.

Yoga doesn't require you to be an acrobat or a vegetarian, nor is it a religion. Religious devotion was never a requirement in the yoga tradition. It simply teaches us to feel responsible for all other life forms in the cosmos. It teaches us to be human. Yoga is really the science of life and death. In the words of the Master, yoga shows us the way to become one with the universe. It teaches us how to recognize ourselves, and it allows us to learn about ourselves physically, emotionally, and spiritually. It helps us recognize how we react to our surroundings. And in fact, there is no difference between us and the world around us. The distinction is artificial.

The belief that we are all different and all have distinct identities is a big illusion. For instance, there is no such thing as a lifeless being, since all beings move and contain energy. Life means energy—even people are made up of energy. Energy means strength. Energy is light, sound, warmth, and coldness. Yoga allows us to discover our innate energies. This gives us strength to help ourselves and the universe, because we possess the qualities of our Creator. With these qualities, I welcome you warmly.

Important Note

The material in this book is intended to provide information about yoga exercises for the body and face that promote a healthier physique and a younger facial appearance. Every effort has been made to provide accurate and dependable information. The contents of this book have been compiled through professional research and in consultation with professionals. However, professionals have differing opinions, and some of the information in this book may become outdated; therefore, the publisher, author, and editors, as well as the professionals quoted in the book cannot be held responsible for any error, omission, or dated material. The authors and publisher assume no responsibility for any outcome of applying the information in this book. Follow the instructions closely. Note that no one should be forced to assume any physical positions that causes them pain or discomfort. If you have questions concerning your exercise program or the application of the information described in this book, please consult a qualified yoga professional.

Acknowledgments

First, I want to thank God for His goodness and blessings.

I would like to thank my children Marilyn "Aileen" and Edwin, Elizabeth "Bette" and Tony, Maria "Meloy" and Julio, and Jesus "Tres" and Emily, who make me happy and proud; my one-of-a-kind grandchildren Winona, Mico, Miyo, Jezie, Ren, and Milo, who give me peace and joy; my honorable teacher and life partner, my husband Adnan "Ananda" Siddviho Çabuk, who walks with me on the path to truth and always supports me with love and devotion; my editor, Seda Darcan Çiftçi, who did an excellent job preparing this book for publication, together with Muhammet Çiftçi, who helped me make this project a reality; my friends, the photographers Ali Kabaş and Mehmet and Feza Acar, who spent many patient and skillful hours working on this job; Hatice Dursun, and all of the other Kaknüs publishing employees who did a wonderful job with the graphics; the staff of Orlanda Publishing of Germany for their efforts in sharing my book with the European side of the world; and last but not the least the great people at Hunter House of California for their efforts in spreading this knowledge to all English-speaking nations, for the knowledge in this book is a key to a healthier, happier, and more-youthful lifestyle.

I would also like to thank everyone who took part in the "Beauty and Face Yoga" program—all those people who use it regularly and successfully, and who inspired me to collect my experience in this book and share it with you.

Let your flesh and your bones be made of love
let every breath be filled with love
your whole being wrapped in love
be love itself!
for where there is love, there is peace.

How Does Yoga for a Beautiful Face Work?

A person's beauty is conveyed by the energy he or she projects. This energy cannot be seen with the naked eye, because emotions also play an important role here. We instinctively recognize the personality and habits of a person by the beauty of his or her energy, which becomes clearer the more it is developed.

Yoga for a Beautiful Face is a concept based on experiences and exercises that will help you learn to be more intensely aware of yourself. It aims for a conscious improvement of your physical, emotional, and spiritual health that takes your current circumstances into account. The most important thing is that you can use this concept to take full advantage of all your options.

Just remember: Physical attractiveness is only part of our outward appearance. It is not enough just to take care of yourself on the surface—we can only grow more content and more beautiful if we take care of our inner values as well.

Growing more beautiful as we age is an art unto itself. In order to accomplish this, we need to get to know ourselves, our various facets. And we should remember that our environmental influences and habits also affect our appearance.

Yoga for a Beautiful Face is not a temporary trend or a simple exercise regimen that you can learn in a few hours. It is a way of life that will naturally make you more youthful. If you do these exercises, they will give you a young, healthy appearance—for the rest of your life. Thus, beauty yoga requires a holistic approach. I realize that in reading this book you may be mainly interested in preventing wrinkles and facial sagging, so I'll start with the information about the facial exercises. Once you have learned and mastered these exercises, though, you should also read the pages that follow. I recommend seeing the *Yoga for a Beautiful Face* program as an integrated approach and practicing it in its entirety to help you reach your goal.

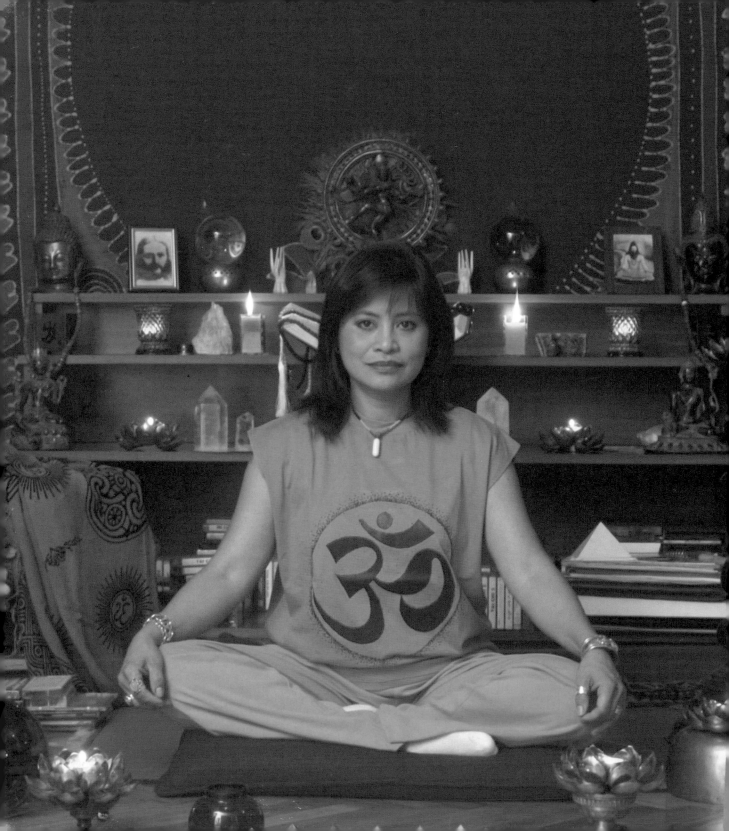

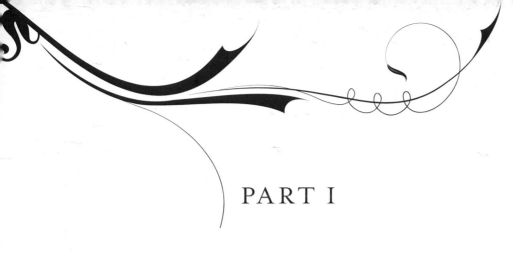

PART I

Yoga for a Beautiful Face

Aging is inevitable, but to age healthily and gracefully is preferable and possible.

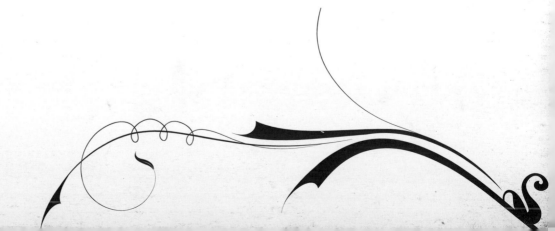

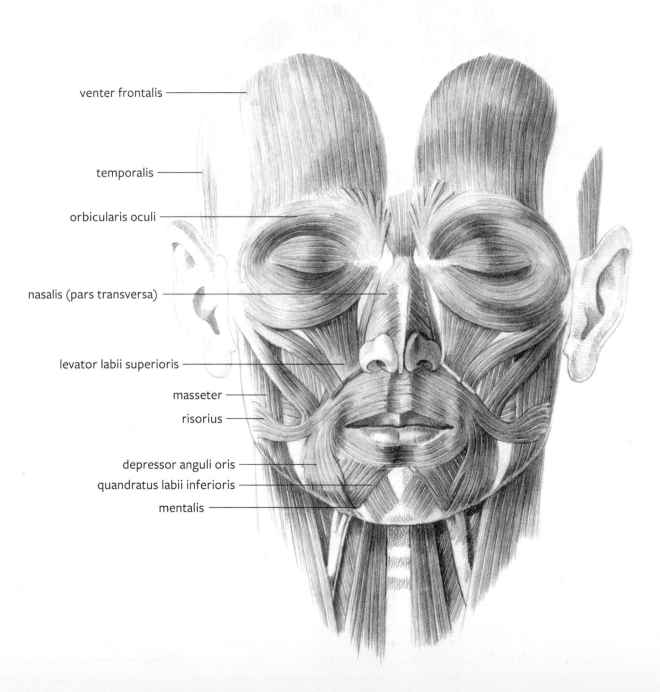

venter frontalis

temporalis

orbicularis oculi

nasalis (pars transversa)

levator labii superioris

masseter

risorius

depressor anguli oris

quandratus labii inferioris

mentalis

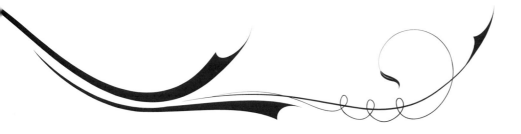

Facial Exercises

Please note! While doing these facial and whole-body exercises, be sure to breathe correctly. Always remember that breath is our source of life.

Every individual cell requires oxygen, especially our facial muscles. You need sufficient oxygen to get the best possible results from these exercises, so I recommend that you read the "Breathing Exercises" section starting on page 53 before starting the other exercises. During the exercises, pay attention to the following things:

1. Before starting a particular exercise, breathe out, then breathe in through your nose, hold your breath for 5 seconds, and breathe out again.
2. Take a deep breath, assume the appropriate exercise position, and hold both the position and your breath for 10 seconds. When you return to the starting position, slowly breathe out. Between exercises, always take a deep breath, hold it for 5 seconds, and then slowly breathe out.
3. Repeat each exercise 3 times. Exceptions to this are the Forehead Massage (see page 6), the eye exercises (see Outer Eye Muscles on page 22, Musculature of the Eyes on page 38, and Eye Wrinkles on page 40), Rolling a Pencil (see page 28), and Lifting a Spoon (see page 30).
4. Do all facial exercises in front of a mirror.
5. If an exercise requires you to move your facial skin in such a way that causes your skin to wrinkle, either do not continue the exercise or modify it as needed.
6. After each exercise, completely relax your muscles for 1 to 2 minutes before moving on. This allows for increased blood circulation in that area and also allows the muscles to rest and become more resilient.
7. For areas that need more work, like a double chin, do the appropriate exercises 6 days a week, 3 times a day. On the 7th day, take a break from the exercises to let your face recover.

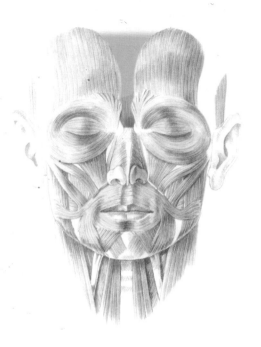

Forehead Massage

Relaxing the facial muscles

- ⊰ Before beginning the exercise, breathe out. Then breathe in through your nose, hold your breath for 5 seconds, and slowly breathe out again.

- ⊰ Using both middle fingers, gently tap your forehead between your eyebrows (the "third eye"), all the way up to your hairline.

- ⊰ Continue breathing in and out normally as you do the exercise for 2 minutes, gently tapping your third eye approximately 100 times.

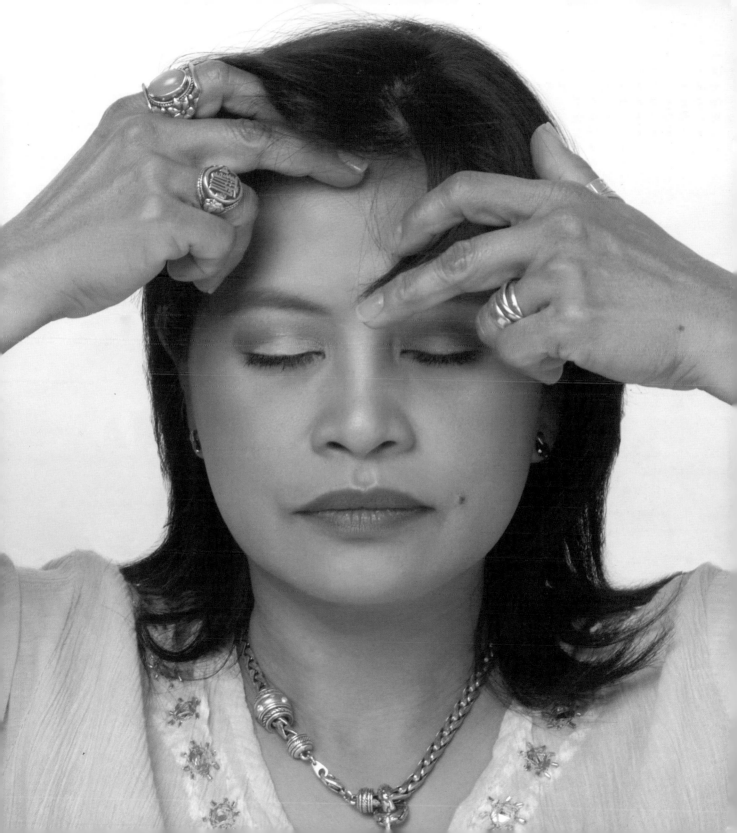

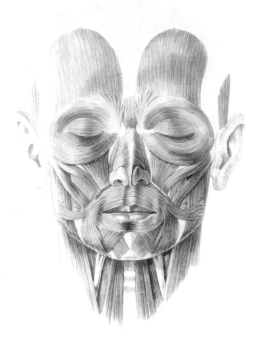

Pulling the Eyebrows Upward

Strengthening the forehead muscles
and the muscles of the upper eyelids

- Before beginning the exercise, breathe out. Then breathe in through your nose, hold your breath for 5 seconds, and slowly breathe out again.

- Place the base of the palms of your hands directly on top of your eyebrows and press your eyebrows upward and to the sides.

- During the exercise, breathe in and feel the tension in your eyebrows as you try to look toward your chest, and then draw your brows together.

- Hold your breath for 10 seconds and stay in this position. As you slowly breathe out, remove your hands from your face.

- Repeat the exercise 3 times.

- Remember to breathe in and hold your breath for 5 seconds between each repetition and then breathe out slowly.

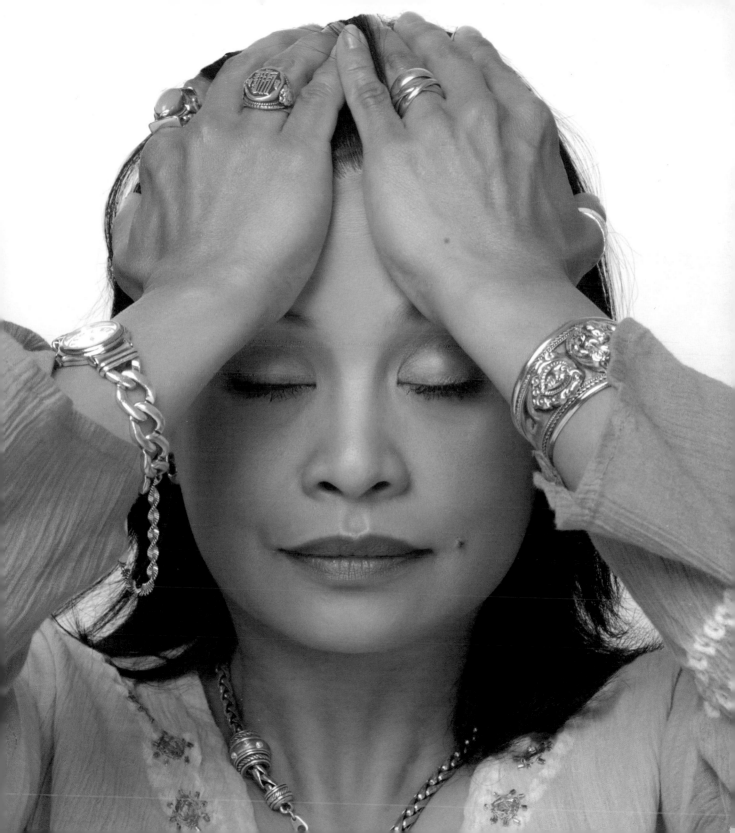

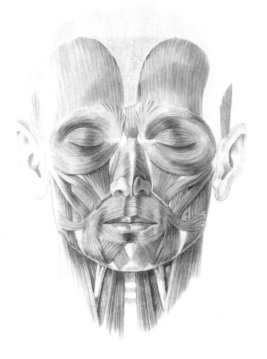

Forehead Wrinkles

Strengthening the
forehead muscles

- Before beginning the exercise, breathe out. Then breathe in through your nose, hold your breath for 5 seconds, and slowly breathe out again.

- Place the tips of your pinky fingers between your eyebrows and the pads of your thumbs on the outer ends of your eyebrows. Pull your eyebrows simultaneously up and to the sides. Make sure that doing this doesn't create any wrinkles.

- Place your other fingertips on your forehead just under your hairline, and use them to pull your forehead muscles and eyebrows upward.

- Breathe in deeply; from this position, look downward. Feel the tension in your eyelids.

- Pull your eyebrows together. Hold this position and your breath for 10 seconds, then breathe out.

- Raise your eyebrows upward again without changing the position of your fingers.

- Repeat the exercise 3 times.

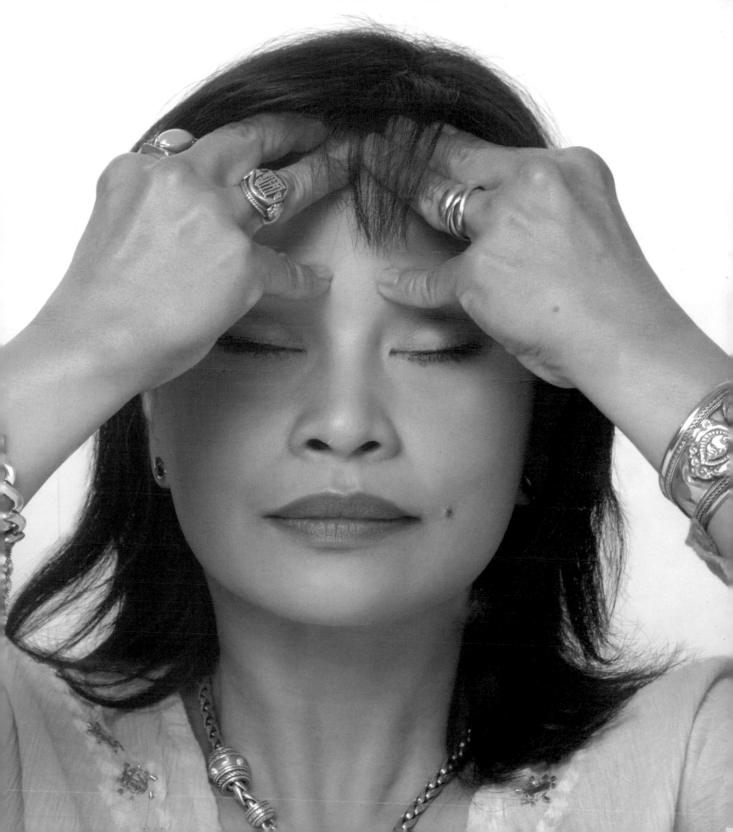

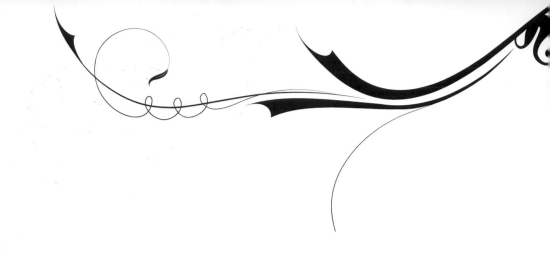

Let your life be that of a rose.
In silence, it speaks the language of fragrance.

Babaji Nagaraj
Founder of Kriya yoga

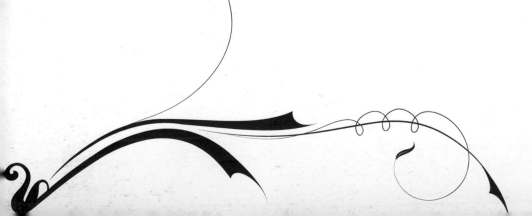

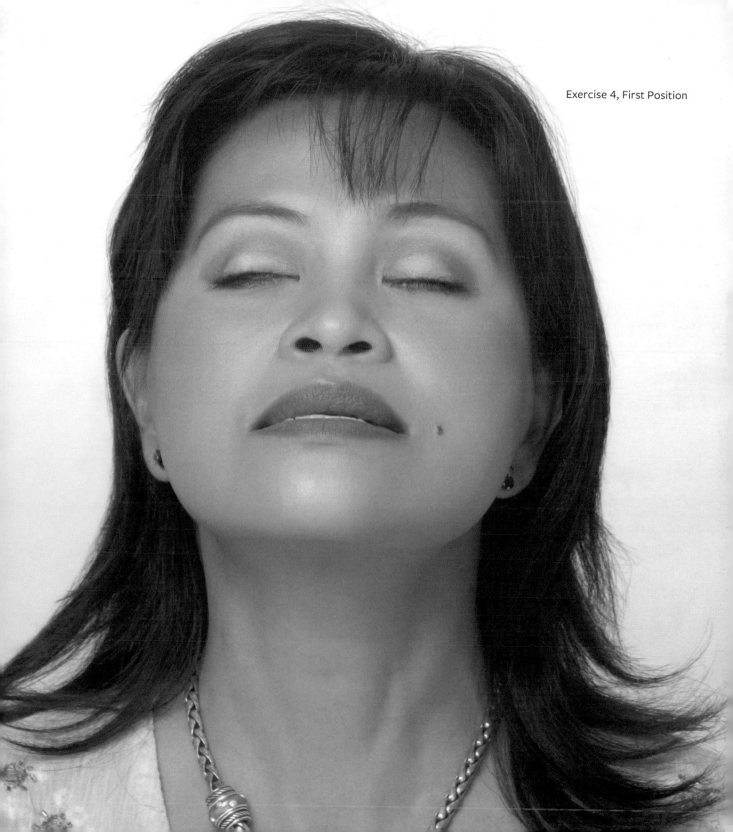

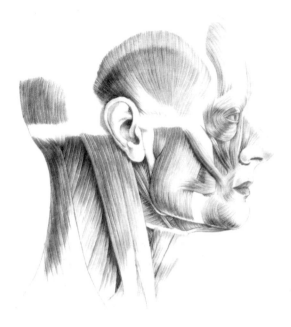

Neck Muscles

Tightening the chin
and neck muscles

⇥ Before beginning the exercise, breathe out. Then breathe in through your nose, hold your breath for 5 seconds, and slowly breathe out again.

⇥ Take a deep breath, then do the two positions shown at right:

Note: *If you have health issues relating to your neck or chin, please consult your doctor before doing this exercise.*

Second Position A

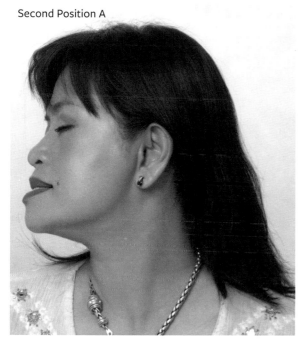

Second Position B

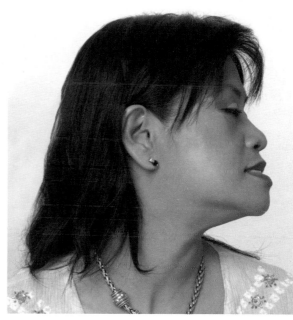

First position (see page 13): With your head in a neutral position (i.e., looking straight ahead), push your chin and lower lip forward. Slowly lean your head back and push your tongue against the roof of your mouth (upper palate). Hold this position for 10 seconds. Meanwhile, use your fingertips to gently tap your chin. Then breathe out and return your head to the starting position.

Second position: Push your chin and lower lip forward. Turn your head to the left. Push your tongue against the roof of your mouth and slightly lean your head back. In this position, pull your chin slightly upward. Hold the position for 10 seconds. Breathe out slowly and return your head to the starting position. Repeat the same sequence on the right side.

Repeat the two positions in this exercise a total of 3 times. Remember to breathe in and out and to relax between repetitions.

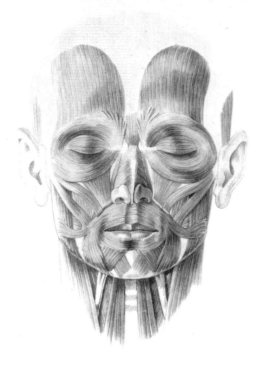

Nasolabial Folds

Smoothing the nasolabial folds
and firming the cheeks

- As shown in the photo, hold your cheek muscles with your thumbs and forefingers, and pull your cheek down slightly (less than a quarter of an inch).

- Take a deep breath. As you do this exercise, open your eyes as wide as possible. Smile broadly to stretch your cheeks as far as you can, first to the sides and then upward, making sure that doing this exercise doesn't create any wrinkles.

- Hold your breath for 10 seconds while holding the position, then breathe out slowly.

- After finishing the exercise, take another deep breath and hold it for 5 seconds. Then breathe out slowly and relax for about 5 seconds.

- Repeat the exercise 3 times.

Note: *If opening your eyes creates wrinkles, do the exercise with your eyes closed. Do not apply any pressure to your cheeks with your fingers. Press the balls of your hands together as shown, and stay in this position.*

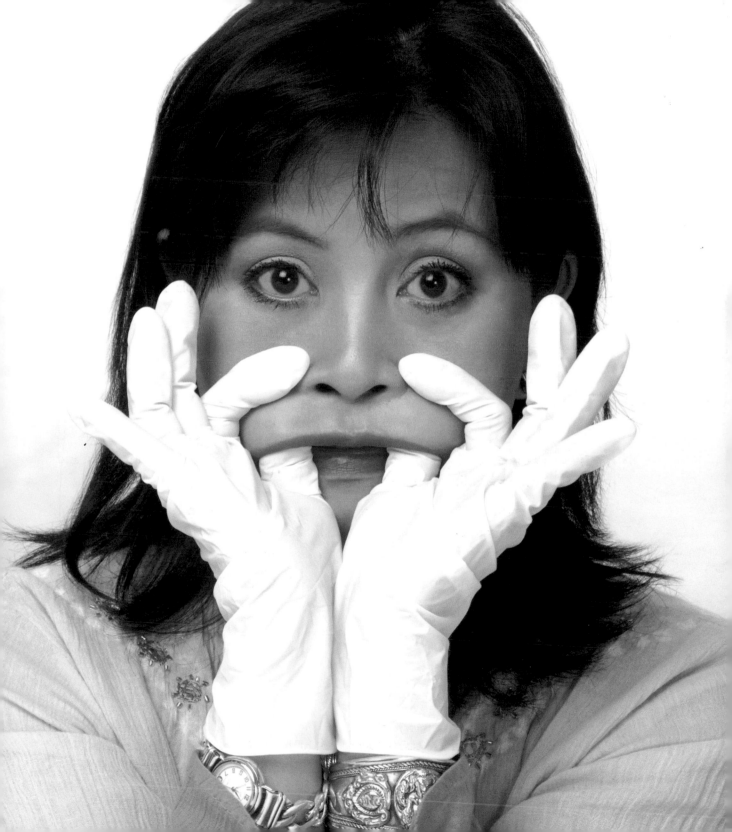

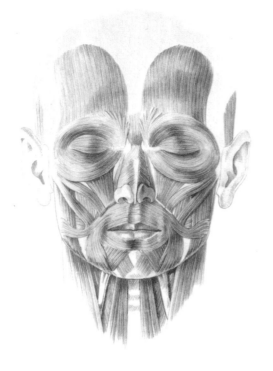

Forehead Muscles

Reducing forehead wrinkles

- Before beginning the exercise, breathe out. Then breathe in through your nose, hold your breath for 5 seconds, and slowly breathe out again.

- Place the tips of three of your fingers on your forehead as shown in the illustration. Place your thumbs on the sides of your head to steady yourself. Use your fingers to pull the skin on your forehead toward your ears.

- Take a deep breath, draw your eyebrows together, and look downward.

- Hold this position and your breath for 10 seconds. Then breathe out slowly.

- Repeat this exercise 3 times. Please remember to breathe in and out and to relax between repetitions.

- As you relax, massage your forehead by slowly tapping it with the tips of your middle fingers to activate blood flow.

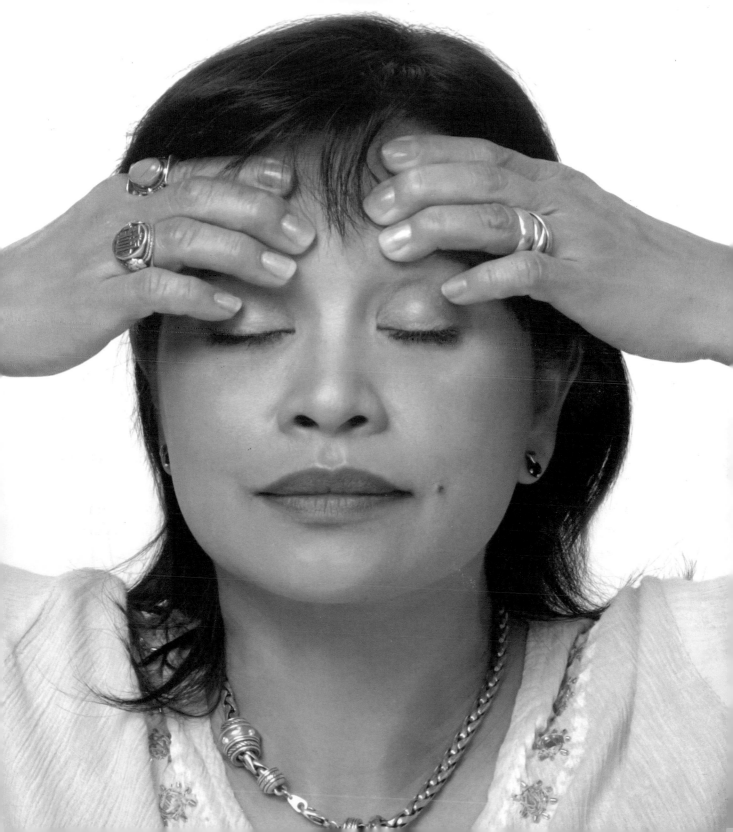

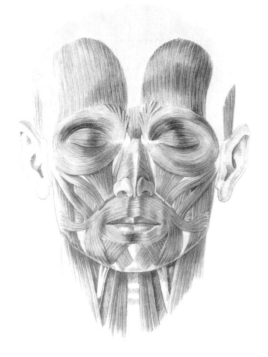

Exercise 7

Major Facial Muscles

Smoothing lip wrinkles and creating fuller lips

- ❧ Before the exercise, take a deep breath. Then open your mouth slightly, roll your lips inward, and while keeping them rolled, move your lips and mouth as if you were making a "U" sound.

- ❧ Open your eyes wide during this exercise!

- ❧ After the "U," make a big "O" with your lips and mouth. Make sure your lips are still pulled in. Smile and pull your cheeks upward, to the sides, and then down. Keep as much tension in your cheeks as you can. Make sure that doing this doesn't create any wrinkles.

- ❧ Hold this position and your breath for 10 seconds, then slowly breathe out.

- ❧ Take another deep breath, hold your breath for 5 seconds, and then breathe out slowly. Relax for about 5 seconds.

- ❧ Repeat this exercise 3 times. Please remember to breathe in and out and to relax between repetitions.

Note: *If opening your eyes creates wrinkles on your forehead, do the exercise with your eyes closed.*

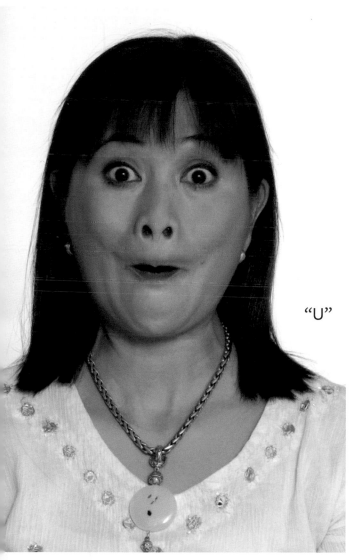

"U"

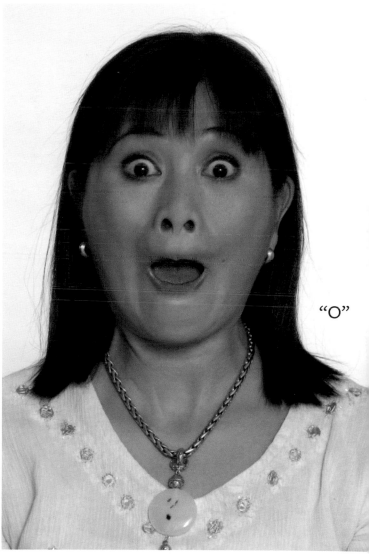

"O"

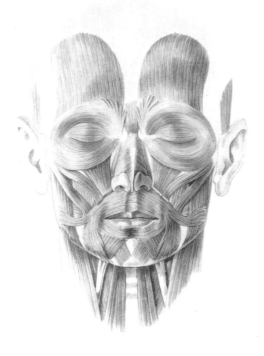

Outer Eye Muscles

Reducing wrinkles
around the eyes

⚞ Open your eyes as wide as you can. Place your index fingers and thumbs on your upper and lower eyelids, palms facing out. Use your middle fingers to pull your forehead muscles upward. Make sure that doing this doesn't create any wrinkles.

First Position

⚞ Breathe deeply before beginning exercise. Looking straight ahead, try to close your eye lids.

⚞ Hold this position and your breath for 10 seconds, then breathe out slowly.

Second Position

⚞ Remain in the starting position. Look upward and try to close your eye lids.

⚞ Stay in this position and hold your breath for 10 seconds, then breathe out slowly.

Third Position

⚞ Remain in the starting position. Look downward and try to close your eye lids.

⚞ Stay in this position, holding your breath, for 10 seconds, then breathe out slowly.

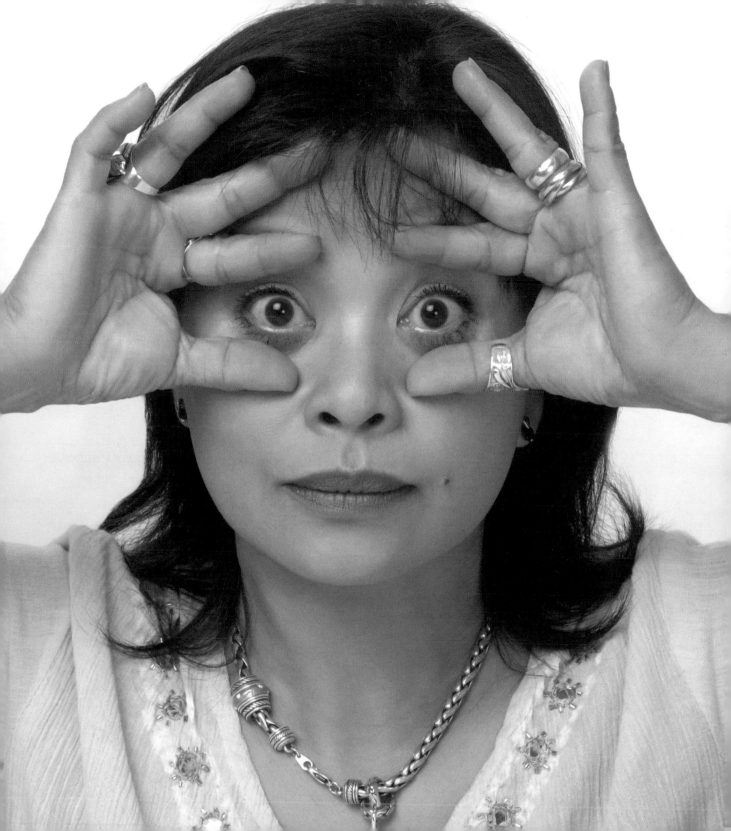

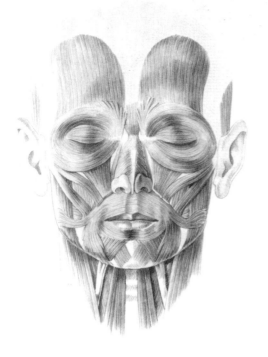

Exercise 9

Musculature of the Mouth (I)

Smoothing out wrinkles around the lips;
a natural way to create fuller lips

- With your thumbs and index fingers, firmly hold the ends of your upper lip, but without pulling it to the sides.

- Before the exercise, take a deep breath.

- From this position, try to purse your lips, creating a gentle resistance.

- Now carefully use your fingers to pull your lips about ¼ inch to each side. Hold this position for 10 seconds, then breathe out slowly.

- In the starting position, take another deep breath. Hold your breath for 5 seconds and then slowly breathe out. Relax for about 5 seconds.

- Repeat the exercise 3 times. Please remember to breathe in and out between repetitions and to relax.

Note: *You should not speak or move the lips for a couple of minutes after performing this exercise. This allows for fuller blood circulation around the lip area and relaxes the lip muscles.*

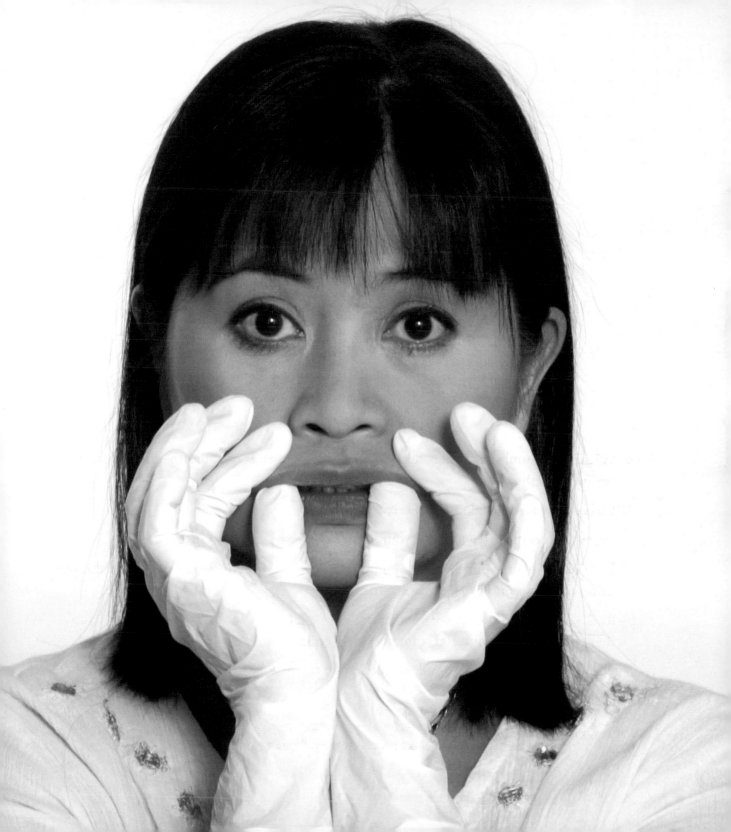

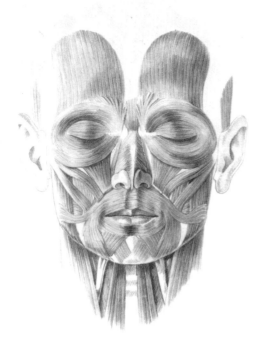

Exercise 10

Firming the Cheeks

Strengthening the lower part
of the cheeks

- Before beginning this exercise, breathe out. Afterward, breathe in through your nose, hold your breath for 5 seconds, and then slowly breathe out again.

- As shown in the illustration, open your mouth slightly; place your index fingers inside your mouth, just below the corners, place your thumbs on the outside of the same spot, pinch the skin lightly, and then gently pull forward and little bit downward.

- From this position, try to draw the lower part of your cheeks to the sides, toward your ears (this looks a bit like an upside-down smile).

- Hold your breath and stay in this position for 10 seconds.

- Repeat the exercise 3 times. Please remember to breathe in and out between the repetitions and to relax.

Note: *Before performing the exercise, draw your head upward and slightly back. Lift your elbows slightly. Make sure that the index fingers inside the mouth do not touch or put pressure on the lower gums and that your other fingers do not touch your lower lip or chin.*

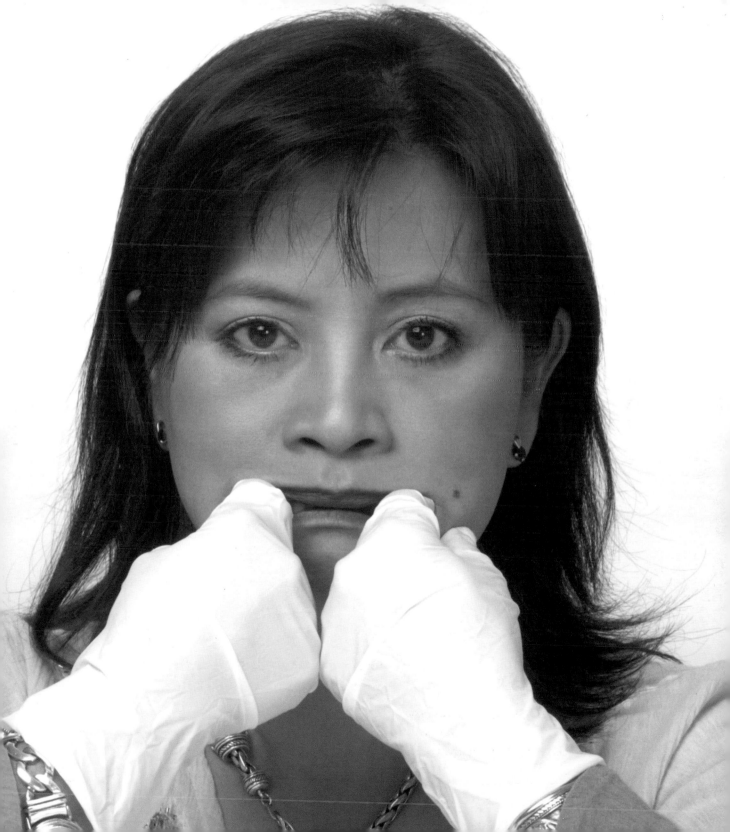

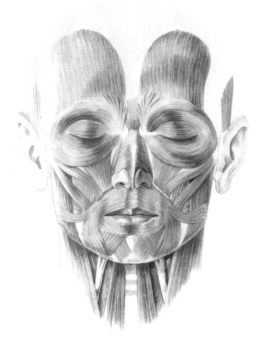

I I

Rolling a Pencil

Strengthening the cheeks, mouth, and neck muscles

⇥ Before beginning this exercise, breathe out. Then breathe in through your nose, hold your breath for 5 seconds, and slowly breathe out.

⇥ As shown in the illustration, hold the pencil with your lips rolled inward.

⇥ Rotate the pencil back and forth with your lips. While your chin is pushed forward, lift your chin slightly and draw your cheeks upward with a slight smile. Hold this position for 2 seconds. Then breathe out slowly and relax your face and chin for 2 seconds.

⇥ Repeat this exercise at least 20 times.

Recommendation: To get faster results, this exercise can be done right after each set of the exercises for the Major Facial Muscles (see Exercise 7 on page 20).

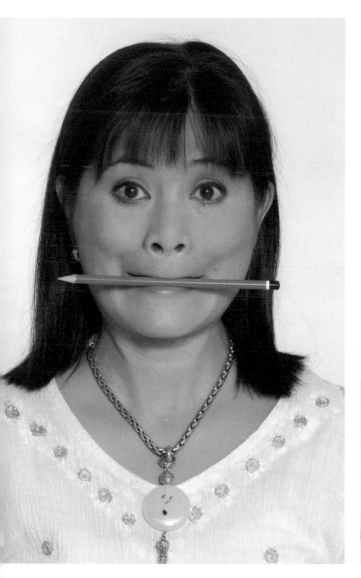
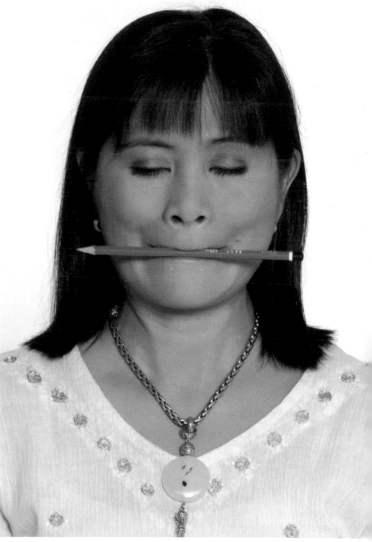

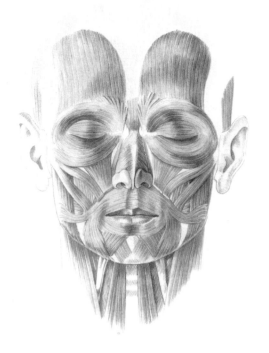

Lifting a Spoon

Strengthening the cheeks, mouth, neck, and pectoral muscles

⇥ Before beginning this exercise, breathe out. Then breathe in through your nose, hold your breath for 5 seconds, and slowly breathe out.

⇥ Roll your lips inward. Place your rolled upper lip on the top side of the spoon's handle and your lower lip on its underside, somewhat farther down.

⇥ Use your lower jaw to lift the spoon as high as you can, and smile to pull your cheeks upward.

⇥ Hold this position for 2 seconds. Afterward, relax your cheek muscles.

⇥ Repeat this exercise at least 20 times.

Recommendation: To get faster results, this exercise can be done right after each set of the exercises for Firming the Cheeks (see Exercise 10 on page 26).

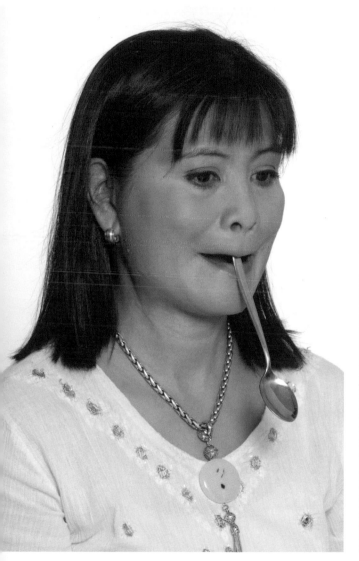
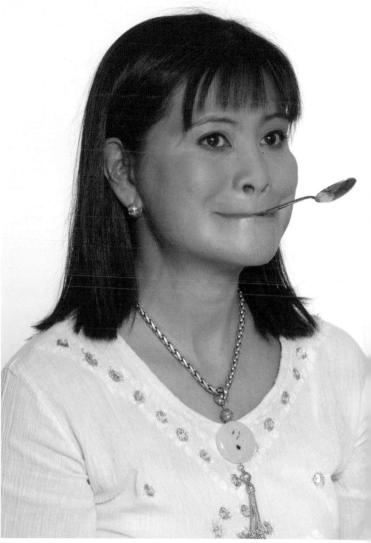

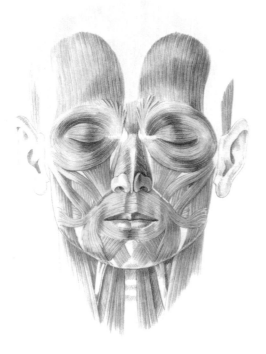

Exercise **13**

Musculature of the Mouth (II)

Tightening the lips, chin, and cheeks

- Before this exercise, take a deep breath. While performing the exercise, open your eyes as wide as possible.

- Open your mouth slightly, and roll your lips inward.

- Form an "A" with your lips, but without saying it aloud. Hold this position for 5 seconds. Close your mouth slightly, but without changing the position. Next, form an "E" with your lips, but without saying it aloud. Hold this position for 5 seconds. After that, close your mouth slightly and form an "I." Hold this position for 5 seconds. Without changing your position, roll your lips inward and form an "O." Hold this position for 5 seconds. Finally, form a "U" with your lips and hold the position for 5 seconds (see page 35).

- Smile as you form each sound, and if you can, flex your cheek muscles in four different directions: upward, to the sides, and downward. Repeat this exercise 3 times.

Note: *If this exercise creates wrinkles in your cheeks, gently place the palms of your hands on the wrinkles, without applying pressure. If opening your eyes wide creates wrinkles on your forehead, you can also keep your eyes closed.*

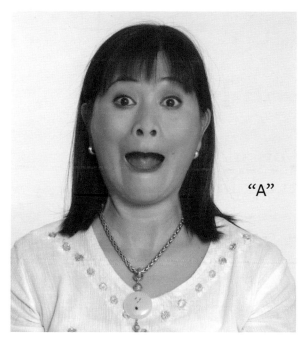

"A"

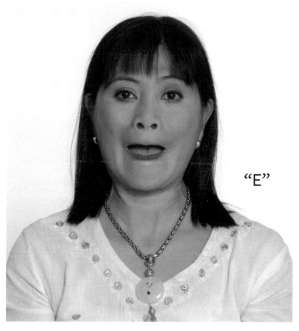

"E"

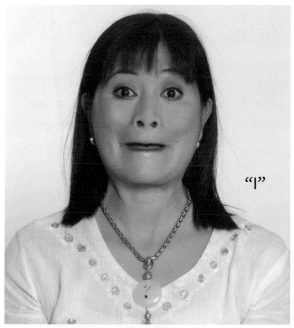

"I"

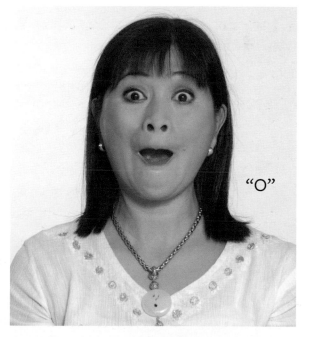

"O"

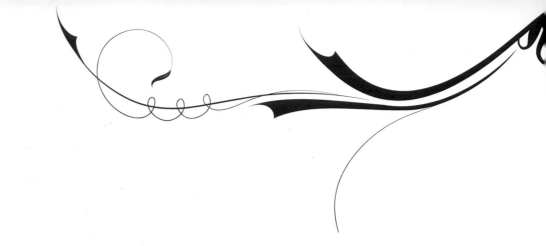

Bad habits can be broken for one's
personal evolution and self-realization.
Only the strong willed and self-confident can achieve this.

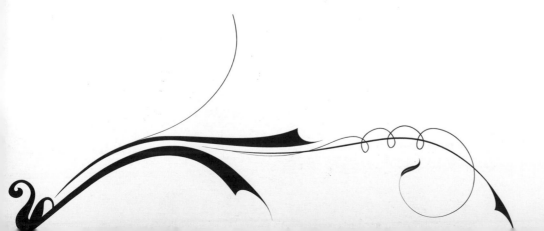

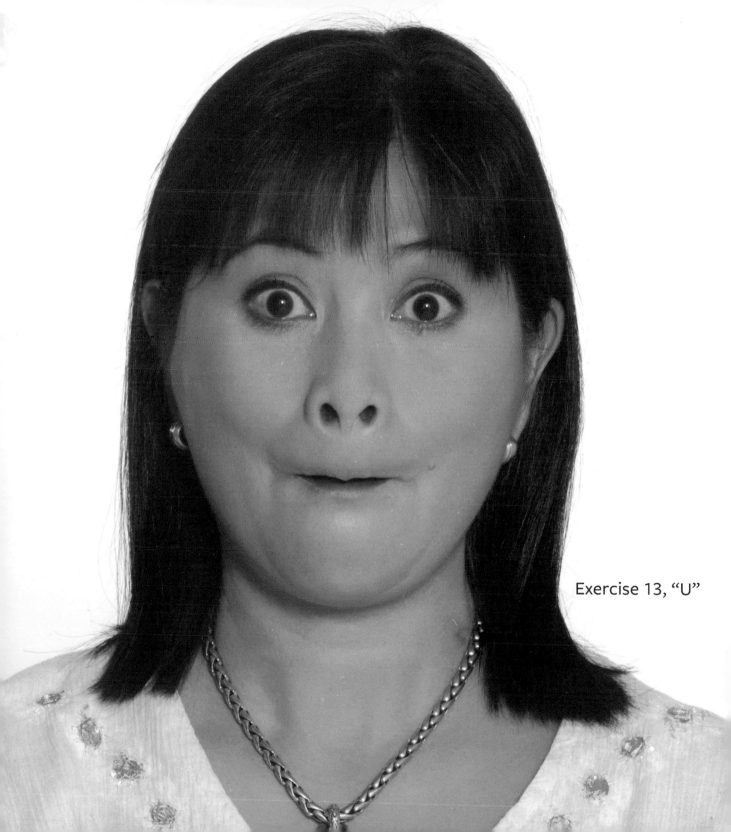

Exercise 13, "U"

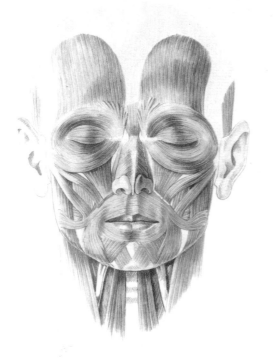

14

Lower Facial Muscles— "Smiling Face"

Strengthening the lower part of the cheeks, the lips, and the musculature of the ear

- Before beginning this exercise, breathe out. Then breathe in through your nose, hold your breath for 5 seconds, and slowly breathe out.

- Your eyes and mouth should remain closed during this exercise to help with concentration.

- Slowly draw the corners of your mouth to the sides in a smile.

- Slowly let your smile grow wider, and draw the corners of your mouth upward as though you were trying to reach your ears. You should be able to feel the tension in your cheeks and lips.

- In this position, hold your breath for 10 seconds and then breathe out.

- Repeat the exercise 3 times.

- Remember to breathe in and out between repetitions and to relax.

Note: *If this exercise creates wrinkles on your cheeks, gently place the palms of your hands on the wrinkles.*

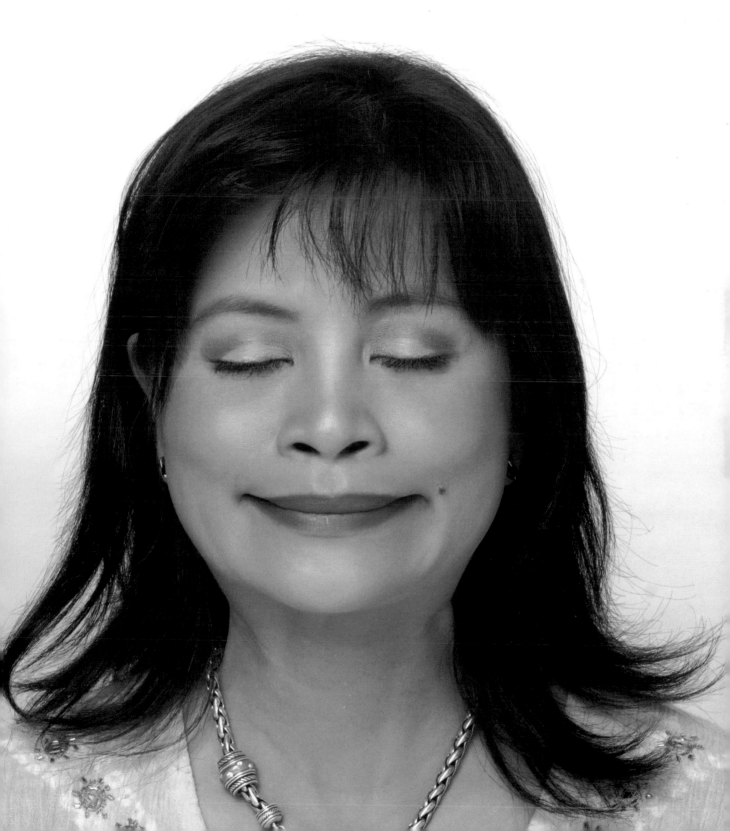

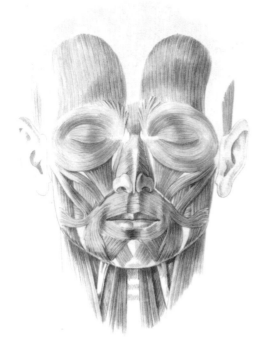

Musculature of the Eyes

Strengthening the circumorbital ring and the eyelids

A. Keep your eyes open as you breathe in and out.

⊰| Look up, and then down; repeat this exercise 3 times.

⊰| Look to the right, and then to the left; repeat this exercise 3 times.

⊰| Look to the top right, and then to the bottom left; repeat this exercise 3 times.

⊰| Look to the top left, and then to the bottom right; repeat this exercise 3 times.

⊰| Roll your eyes clockwise 3 times; then repeat this exercise 3 times rolling your eyes in the opposite direction.

⊰| Blink your eyes. Rub the palms of your hands together to warm them. Then cover your eyes with your palms for 10 seconds. While breathing in, slide your hands outward toward your ears.

⊰| Take a deep breath; hold your breath for 5 seconds, then slowly breathe out. Relax for about 5 seconds.

B. Repeat the exercise, this time with your eyes closed.

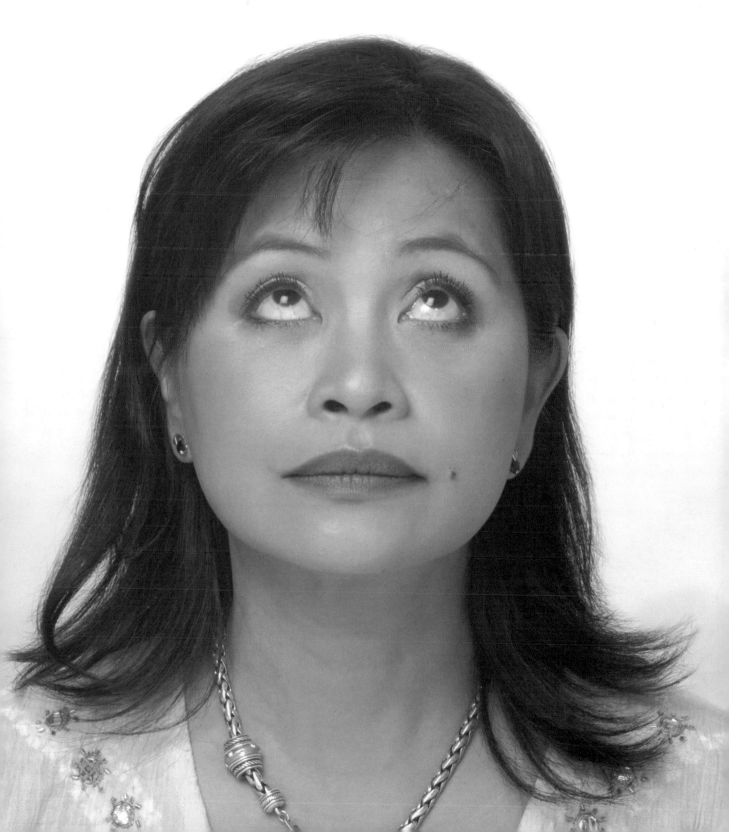

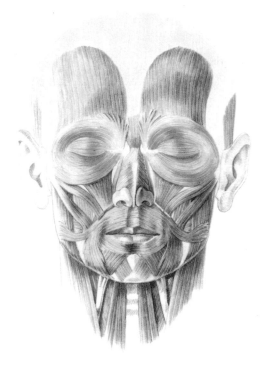

Eye Wrinkles— "Crow's Feet"

❧ Place your thumbs at the outer edges of your eyes. Use your other fingers to push your forehead muscles upward. As you do so, calmly breathe in and out.

❧ Close your eyelids as much as you can, and hold this tension for about 10 seconds.

❧ Look upward without changing the position of your hands, and close your eyelids. Hold your breath in this position for about 10 seconds.

❧ Look downward without changing the position of your hands, and close your eyelids. Hold your breath, and stay in this position for about 10 seconds.

❧ Blink your eyes. Rub the palms of your hands together to warm them, close your eyes, and then cover your eyes with your palms for about 10 seconds. As you breathe out, slide your hands outward toward your ears.

❧ Take a deep breath; hold your breath for about 5 seconds, then slowly breathe out. Relax for about 5 seconds.

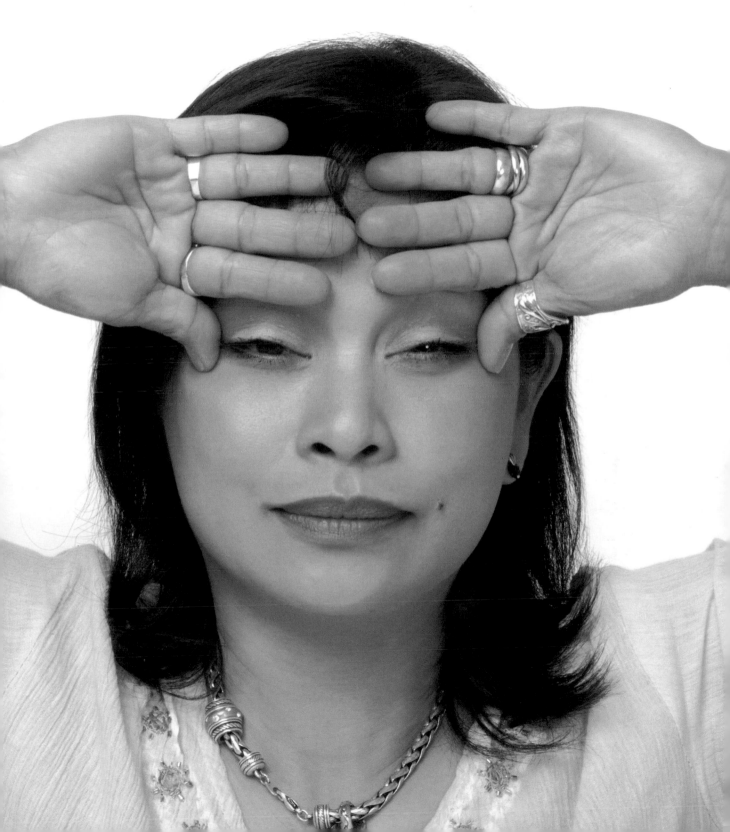

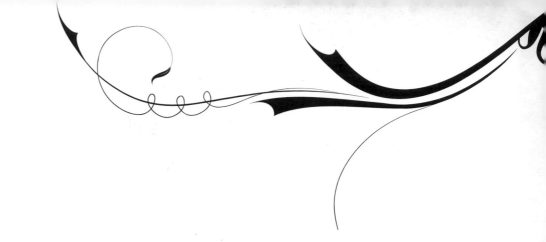

The learning process begins deep within us…
Start by giving up your ego.
If you can do that,
the rest will flow like water.

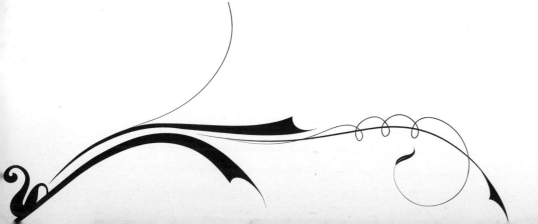

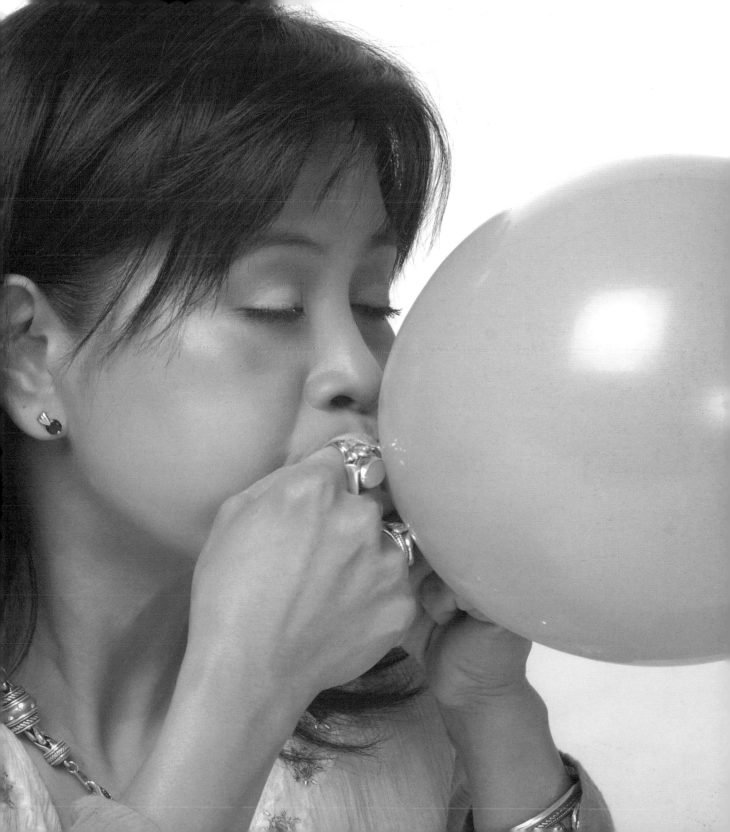

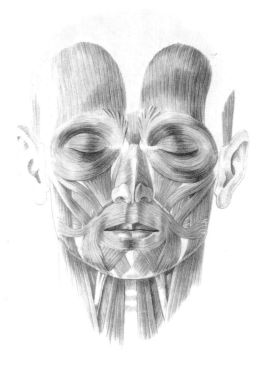

Blowing
up a Balloon

Strengthening the lungs
and facial muscles

☙ Breathe in through your nose and out into the balloon. As you do so, inflate both the balloon and your cheeks as much as possible. Then slowly let the air from the balloon flow back into your mouth. This massages the muscles inside your mouth. Make sure not to inhale or swallow any air from the balloon!

☙ Repeat this exercise 3 times. After doing the exercise, you should not talk or move your face for about 2 minutes.

Note: *For the first week, smokers should only blow the balloon up to the size of an apple. Gradually increase the size of the inflated balloon according to your level of comfort.*

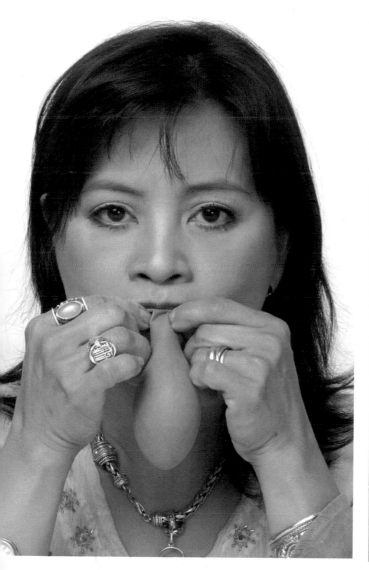

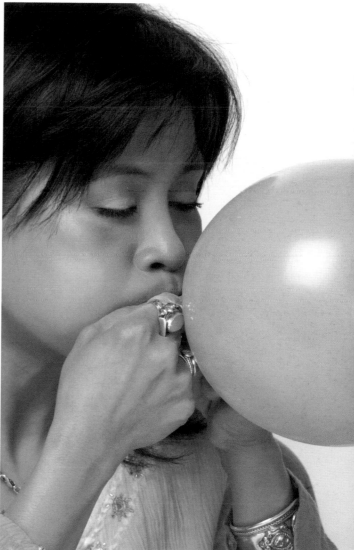

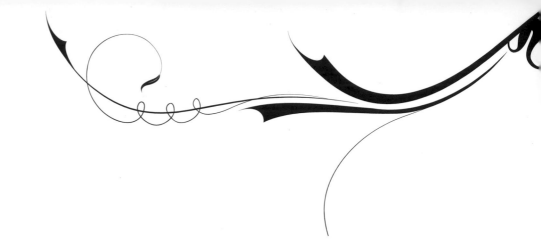

To be humble is a way to reach Nirvana,
for you are nothing but a grain of dust
in the vast universal existence.
You are nothing…nothing!
As from dust you became,
to dust you shall return.

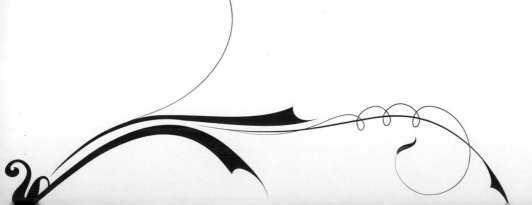

PART II

Yoga for the Rest of Your Body

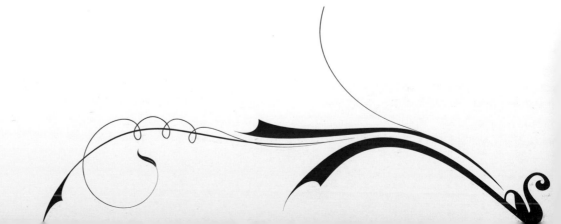

Yoga for a Radiant Presence

The second part of the program, "Yoga for the Rest of your Body," may also be called "Yoga for a Radiant Presence." The second part of the program will help you achieve a healthier lifestyle and a younger appearance and is based on two elements:

1. the five principles of traditional yoga
2. the (healthy) functioning of the three main organs

The Five Principles of Traditional Yoga

The five principles of traditional yoga are proper relaxation, proper breathing, proper nutrition, the proper exercises, and positive thinking.

Proper Relaxation

Proper relaxation creates harmony between the body and the spirit. If we do not practice it, we are blocking the flow of our life energy. If you can practice this form of relaxation at work, for example, you can awaken more energy reserves within yourself. The condition of the spirit is closely linked with the condition of the body. If your muscles are relaxed, your spirit will be, too.

Proper Breathing

We can survive for a few weeks without food, but we cannot live longer than a couple of minutes without breathing. The oxygen that we take in with each breath transforms the nutrient molecules in our cells into energy. No matter how much oxygen is in the atmosphere, we can only store as much as our red blood cells need. If there are not enough red blood cells, our bodies cannot take in the necessary amount of oxygen. Thus proper breathing, nutrition, the right exercises, and positive thinking all work together in harmony.

Proper Nutrition

Proper nutrition means that you are taking in the right nutrients. Make sure to give your body foods that contains all the necessary vitamins and minerals that it needs, at the right time, and be aware of the foods you are combining.

Proper Exercises

You should choose exercises that are appropriate for your fitness level and your constitution. If you are starting an exercise program, take your age, weight, height, any physical challenges, and your muscle and bone composition into account.

As with any kind of exercise or athletic activity, such as walking, jogging, swimming, aerobics, dancing, yoga, or Pilates, proper breathing is very important; when we move, our muscles need oxygen to burn energy.

As you can see, the principles of yoga are very closely linked.

Positive Thinking

Try to look at your life in a constructive way, avoiding negative words and thoughts, and you will notice that your existence takes on a different, more orderly shape. In order to practice this "system of positive thinking," try to keep the following five lower emotions under control: anger, envy, hatred, fear, and egotism.

Start with the emotion/attitude that you have the most trouble with, and try to keep it under control for one year. With this approach, you can more or less gain control over all five of these emotions within five years and more easily practice positive thinking.

The Importance of the Three Main Organs

The three main organs of the human body described next should be healthy and functional in order for the "yoga for a radiant appearance" program to be fully effective.

1. Lungs: With the right kind of breathing, you can use your lungs to their full capacity.
2. Intestines: Special exercises can help support the performance of your intestines and bowels.
3. Spinal column (and brain): Targeted exercises can strengthen these areas.

If you want to apply this knowledge and these principles, make sure these three main organs are working well. In the following pages, you will find a chapter with appropriate exercises. After that, I give recommendations for a daily exercise and health regime. This program also has a positive effect on the beauty and face yoga exercises described previously.

The Daily Exercise Program

Exercises that are best done before breakfast:

Exercises for a Healthy Body

⇥ Yoga breathing (belly and chest breathing): Do repetitions in sets of 3. (This can be done in bed or on the floor.)

⇥ Sideways bellows breathing: 6 repetitions in sets of 3.

⇥ Abdominal exercises: Do repetitions in sets of 4.

⇥ Spinal exercises: Do repetitions in sets of 3.

Internal and External Cleansing

1. For internal cleansing: Add 1 teaspoon of lemon juice and a tiny pinch of salt to a glass of lukewarm water and drink it. This process cleanses your mouth, esophagus, and digestive tract.

2. For external cleansing: I suggest taking lukewarm showers every day. And once a week, before taking a bath, dissolve 10 tablespoons of sea salt in 1½ liters of water and slowly pour it over yourself from head to toe. Make sure the entire body—including the hair roots, fingers, and toes—is soaked for 1 minute. Then immediately rinse the whole body with lukewarm water, after which time you may continue to take a normal bath with soap and shampoo. Doing this balances your positive and negative energies, and increases your sense of well-being.

3. After showering, drink a glass of warm water with 1 teaspoon of lemon juice or apple-cider vinegar and 1 teaspoon of honey. If you tend to have heartburn, use lemon juice, since it becomes alkaline during digestion.

4. Yoga exercises for the face: On the face muscle diagram on page 4, mark the areas you want to tone. Do the exercises targeting your problem areas 6 days a week, 3 times a day. On the 7th day, take a break from the exercises to let your face rest.

Before you begin the physical exercises, please read the next section, which explains how to perform the breathing exercises.

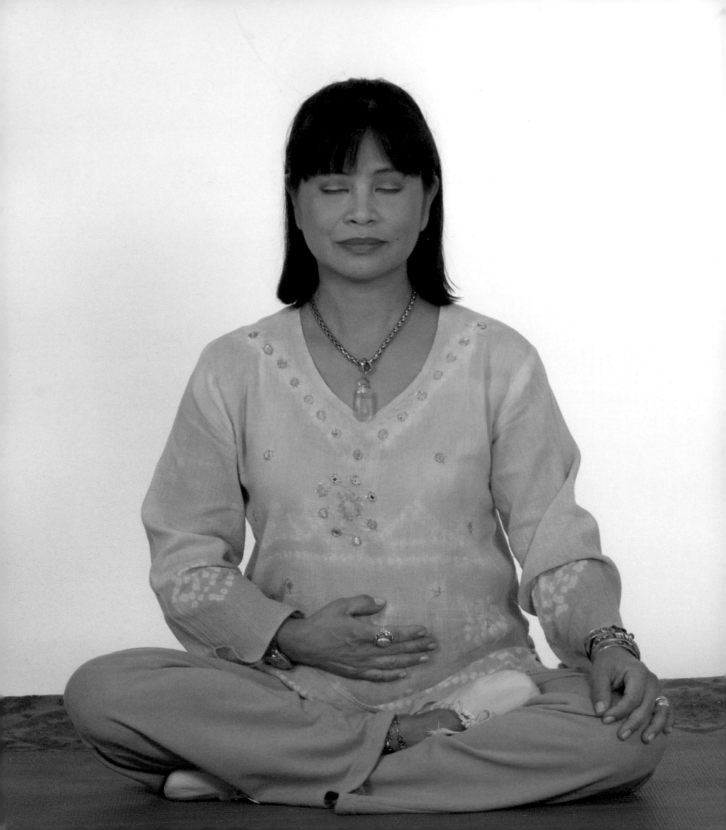

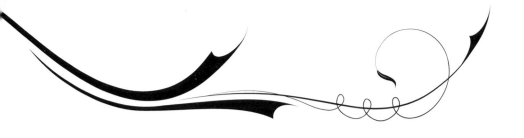

Breathing Exercises

Listen to the sound of silence,
for the answer to everything is within it.

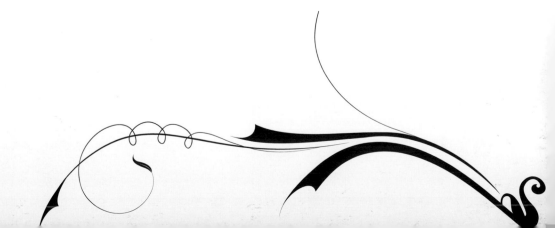

What Is Proper Breathing?

BREATHING IN

BREATHING OUT

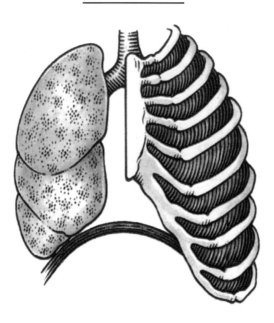
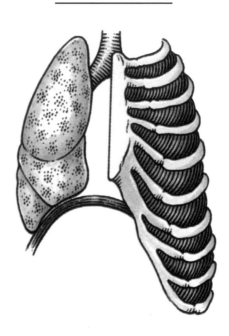

1. As you breathe in through your nose, your belly muscles relax and your belly expands.
2. Air flows through the windpipe into the lungs.
3. The diaphragm is lowered, the lungs are filled with air, and the rib cage expands.

1. As the air flows back out through your nose, your belly muscles contract.
2. This draws the rib cage back together, and the used-up air is exhaled.
3. The diaphragm is drawn upward and the lungs are compressed.

Why Do Yoga Breathing Exercises?

- The yoga exercises create a unity of body and spirit, of the conscious and the subconscious mind.

- The most simple breathing exercise, but also the most important one, is Deep Belly and Chest Breathing (see Breathing Exercise 1 on the next page). Through this exercise, we learn to breathe properly and use our lungs to their full capacity. The exercise provides plenty of oxygen to the body, particularly the brain, along with prana, or "life force."

- Breathing plays a central role in the face yoga exercises, since oxygen is used as soon as the facial muscles are activated.

- If Sideways Bellows Breathing (see Breathing Exercise 2 on page 58) is done correctly, it will purify your entire breathing system, from your airways to your sinuses to your lungs. In other words, even your aura will reflect the good health of your organs.

- This method of breathing enriches the bloodstream with oxygen.

- The exercise strengthens the belly muscles. It gently massages the liver, spleen, pancreas, stomach, and heart, revitalizing the organs and promoting good digestion.

- Yoga breathing enlivens the spirit.

- It improves concentration.

- The third eye may be activated.

- It strengthens the digestive and respiratory systems, stimulates blood circulation, and keeps the nervous system healthy.

Deep Belly and Chest Breathing (Yogic Breathing)

⇥ Lie down on your back and place both hands on your belly.

⇥ Breathe out forcefully, and then slowly take a deep breath. As you breathe in, first extend your belly, then fill your lungs. Feel your rib cage expanding, and slowly draw your shoulders downward. Hold this breath for 5 seconds.

⇥ Breathe out normally, and relax.

⇥ Repeat this exercise 3 times.

Note: *You may experience a slight to medium amount of head spinning or dizziness after this exercise. This is normal, as the brain is getting more oxygen than it usually does, and you will feel better after a few series of breathing exercises.*

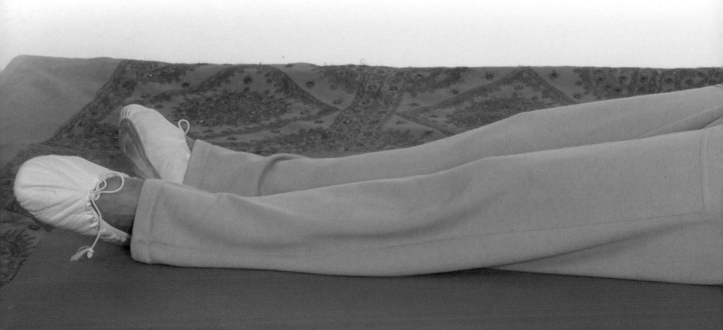

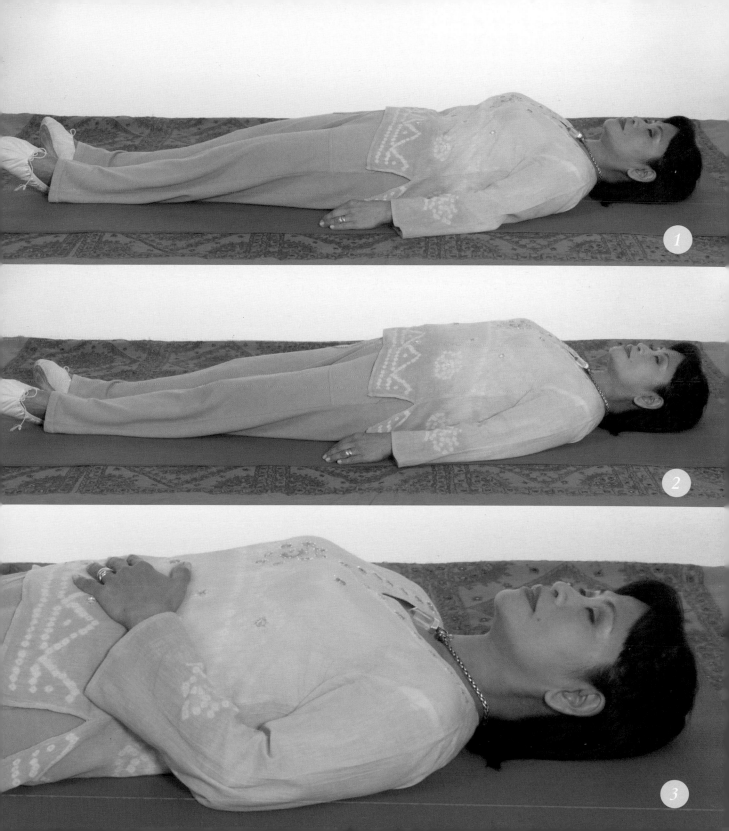

Sideways Bellows Breathing

You should only start doing this breathing exercise once you are sure you are doing the Deep Belly and Chest Breathing from the previous exercise correctly.

- Lie on your left side, as shown in the illustration. Place your right arm on your right hip.

- Make sure your whole spine is as straight as possible.

- As you take a deep breath, push your body forward, and feel your belly expand. As you breathe out, draw your hips and belly back in, hunching your back slightly.

- Repeat this exercise 6 times without interruptions. As you do the exercise, make flowing, snakelike movements and breathe in and out a total of 6 times.

- Finally, lie on your right side and repeat the entire sequence.

- Repeat the entire exercise 3 times.

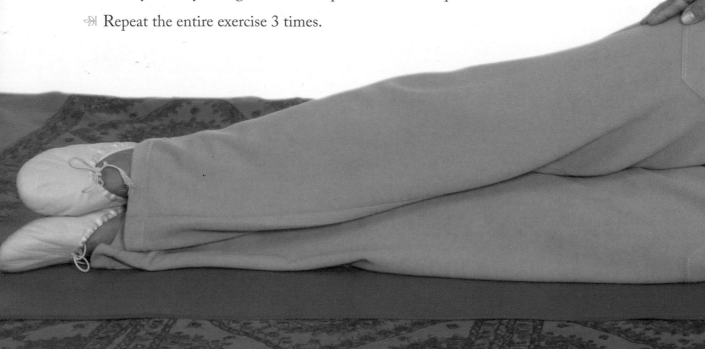

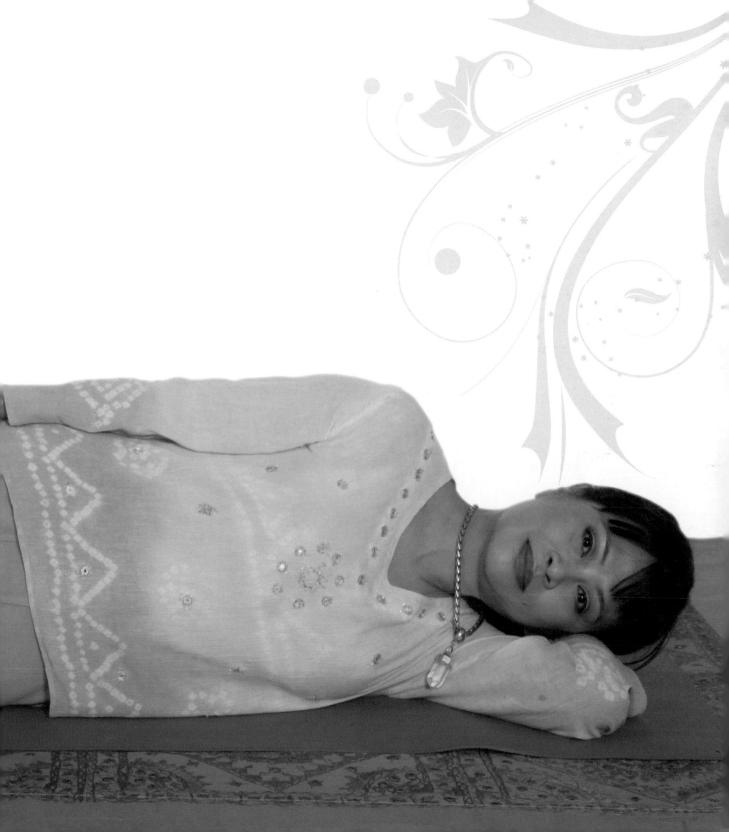

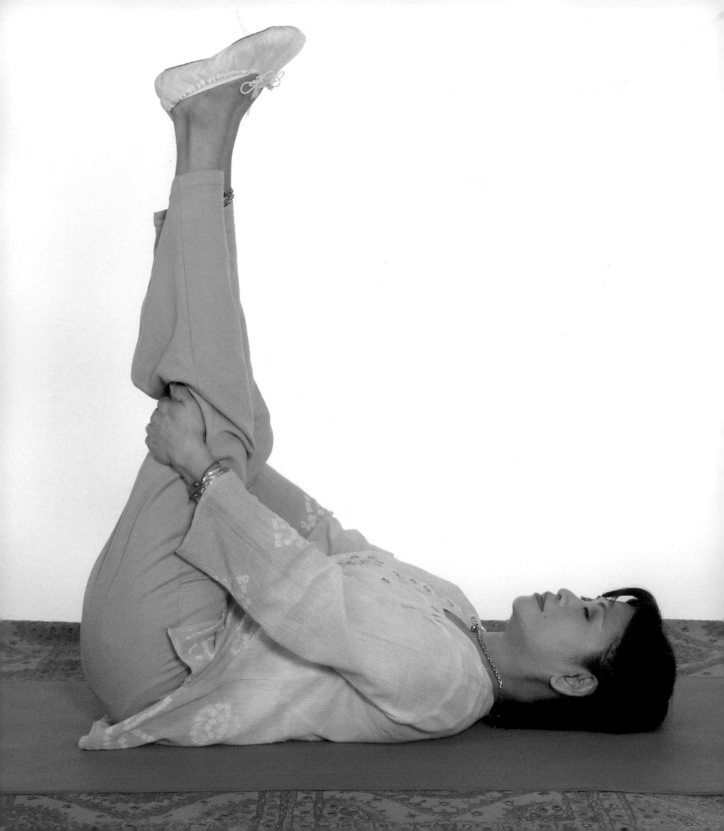

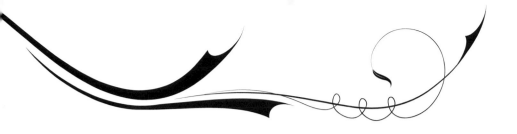

Abdominal Exercises

Events come and go.
This is the wheel of "Maya."
Let the wheel spin around you
without your attachment to any part of it.
Let go of the spokes. Live in the center.
That is "Reality."

Babaji Nagaraj
Founder of Kriya yoga

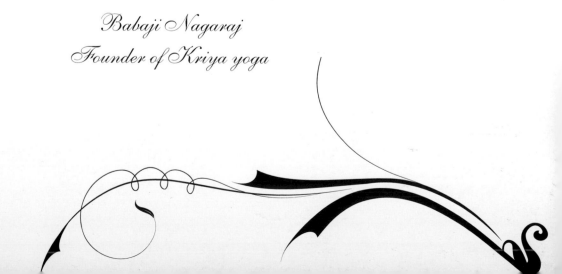

Intestinal Reflex Zones

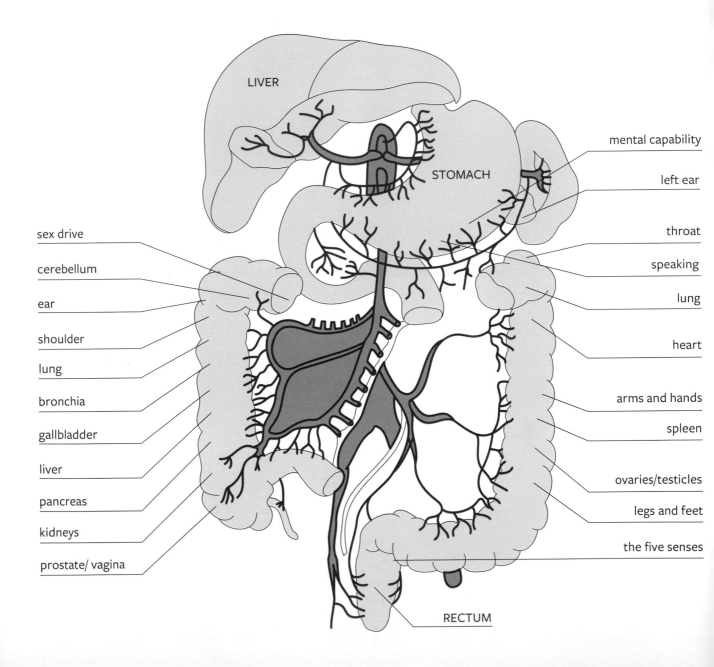

LIVER

STOMACH

mental capability

left ear

throat

speaking

lung

heart

arms and hands

spleen

ovaries/testicles

legs and feet

the five senses

sex drive

cerebellum

ear

shoulder

lung

bronchia

gallbladder

liver

pancreas

kidneys

prostate/ vagina

RECTUM

Activating Your Intestines to Improve Your Health and Beauty

Did you know that the intestine is like a mirror that reflects the various parts of our body?

The illustration at left shows which areas of the intestine affect which body parts.

If our intestinal function is disrupted, we not only lose our vibrancy and our attractiveness, but are also at risk for serious health problems such as colon cancer.

On the following pages, I provide you with four illustrated exercises to regulate intestinal peristalsis (the involuntary contractions required for your bowels to move waste). Doing these exercises regularly will help to make your bowel movements regular and will increase your vibrancy.

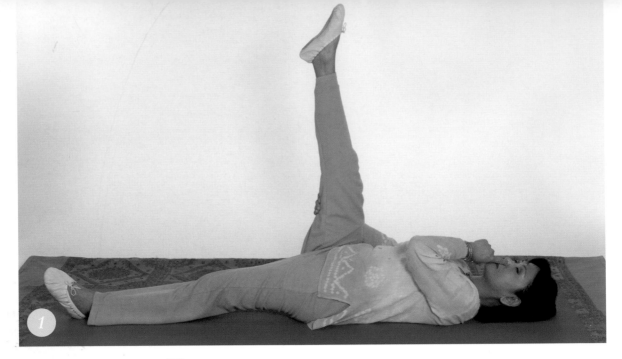

Abdominal Exercise I

- ✦ Lie down on your back in a comfortable position (preferably on the floor with a yoga mat or thick blanket.)

- ✦ Before starting this exercise, massage your belly. Use base of the palm of your right hand and start on the right side just below the belly. Massage upward using circular motions as you breathe in, then move to the middle, to the left side, and downward as you breathe out. Do this massage sequence 3 times.

- ✦ Use your left hand to close your left nostril. As you take a deep breath through your right nostril, grasp your right leg firmly, just below the knee, with your right hand. Bend this leg and gently pull it in toward your body.

- ✦ Pull your knee close to your chest as you slowly breathe out.

- ✦ Do the deep belly and chest breathing exercise 3 times in this position.

- ✦ Straighten your right leg as you take another deep breath.

- ✦ Slowly place your leg back on the ground as you breathe out.

- ✦ Repeat the exercise with your left leg, using your right hand to close your right nostril.

- ✦ This exercise can be viewed as a set, and should be done 3 sets at a time.

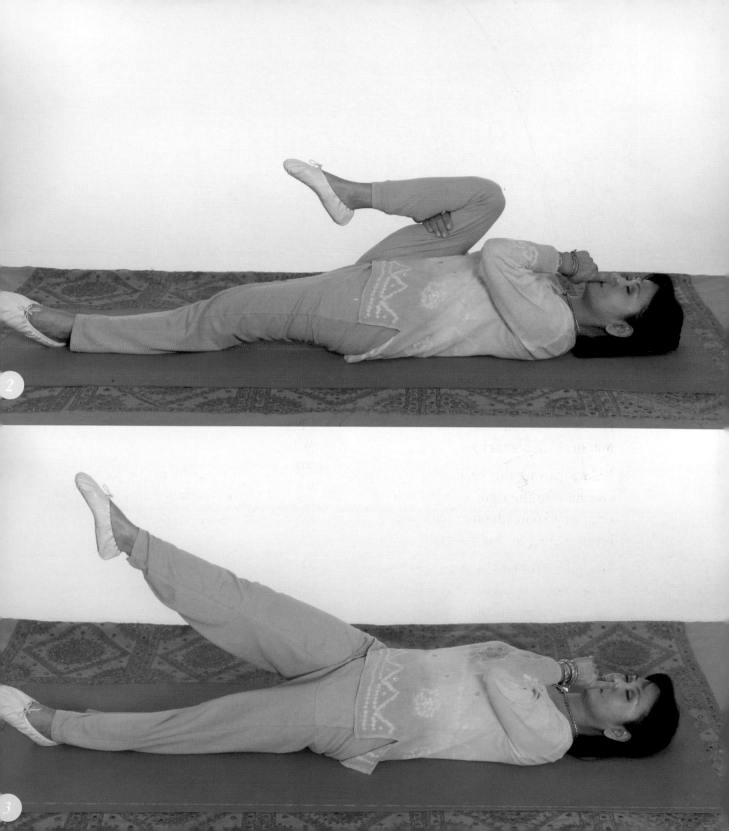

2

3

Abdominal Exercise 2

⋈ Lie on the floor. Lift both legs at a right angle to your torso as you take a deep breath.

⋈ Clasp your hands below your knees and as you breathe out, bend your knees and draw your legs in toward your belly while pressing your back into the floor.

⋈ Do the Deep Belly and Chest Breathing exercise (see page 56) 3 times in this position.

⋈ Now breathe in, and roll over onto your right side. Breathe out, and roll onto your left side. Repeat this 3 times. (Doing this activates the reflex points on the back for the intestines and relaxes the spine.)

⋈ Come back to the middle, breathe in, and stretch your legs up to the ceiling.

⋈ As you breathe out, lower your legs back onto the floor.

Notes:
1. If you have back problems, keep your knees bent as you lower your legs and feet back onto the floor.
2. Contract the abdominal muscles when lowering the legs. Doing this prevents you from feeling any discomfort in the lumbar region of the spine

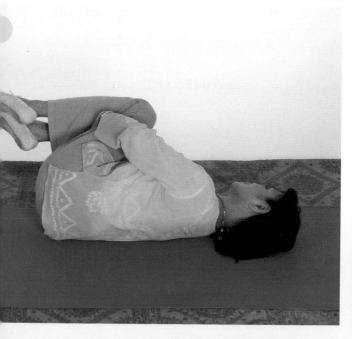

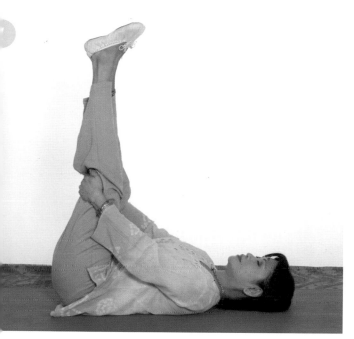

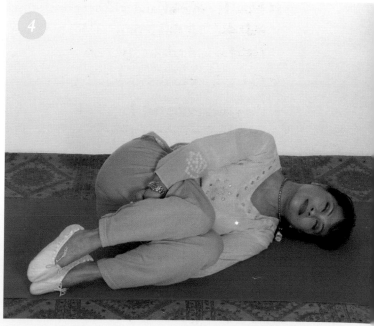

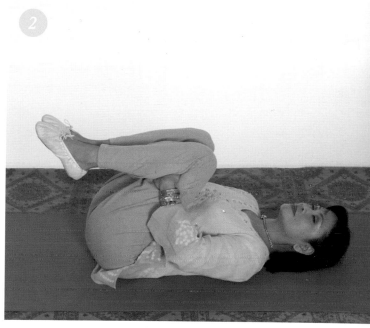

Abdominal Exercise 3

⊁| While still lying down on your back, raise your bent knees to the sides, breathe in calmly, and put the soles of your feet together just above your belly.

⊁| Grasp your feet with both hands, keeping your elbows between your knees.

⊁| As you breathe out, gently pull your feet as far as you can toward your chest.

⊁| Do the deep belly and chest breathing exercise 3 times in this position.

⊁| Take another breath, and roll over onto your right side. Breathe out, and roll onto your left side. Repeat this 3 times.

⊁| Once you are back in the middle, breathe in and stretch your legs up toward the ceiling.

⊁| As you breathe out, slowly lower your legs back onto the floor.

Notes:
1. If you have back problems, keep your knees bent as you lower your legs and feet back onto the floor.
2. Contract the abdominal muscles when lowering the legs. Doing this prevents you from feeling any discomfort in the lumbar region of the spine

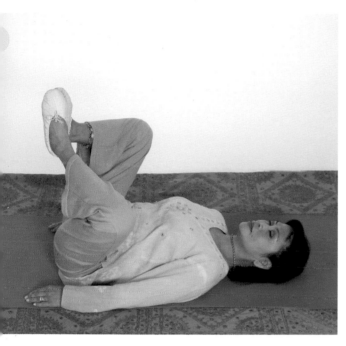

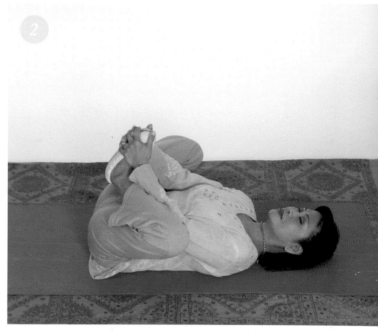

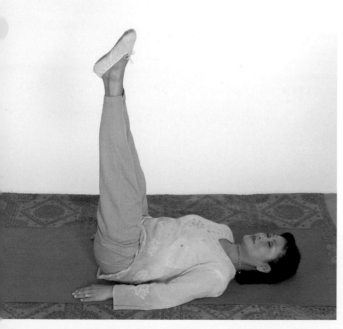

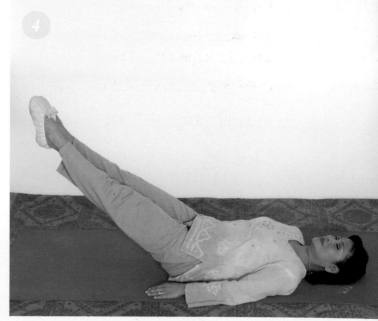

Abdominal Exercise 4

- While still lying down on your back, raise your bent knees to the sides and keep them shoulder-width apart.

- Take a deep breath, pulling your knees in closer to your shoulders. Your calves should be parallel to the ground.

- Grasp your feet with your hands, making sure that your arms are on the outsides of your knees.

- Pull your feet in toward you, and bring your knees to your chest as you breathe out.

- Do the Deep Belly and Chest Breathing exercise (see page 56) 3 times in this position.

- Take another breath, and roll over onto your right side. Breathe out, and roll onto your left side. Repeat this 3 times.

- Once you are back in the middle, breathe in and stretch your legs up to the ceiling.

- As you breathe out, slowly place your legs back on the floor.

Notes:
1. If you have back problems, start and finish the exercise with your knees bent.
2. Contract the abdominal muscles when lowering the legs. Doing this prevents you from feeling any discomfort in the lumbar region of the spine.

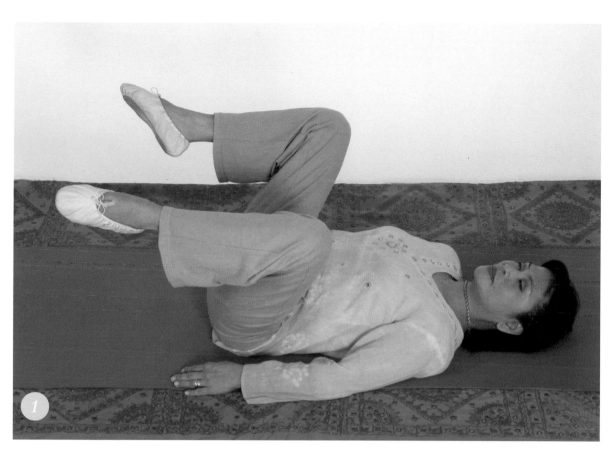

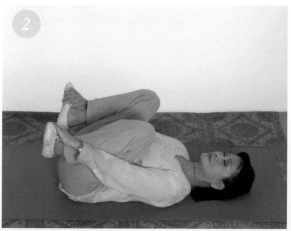

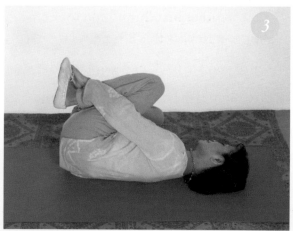

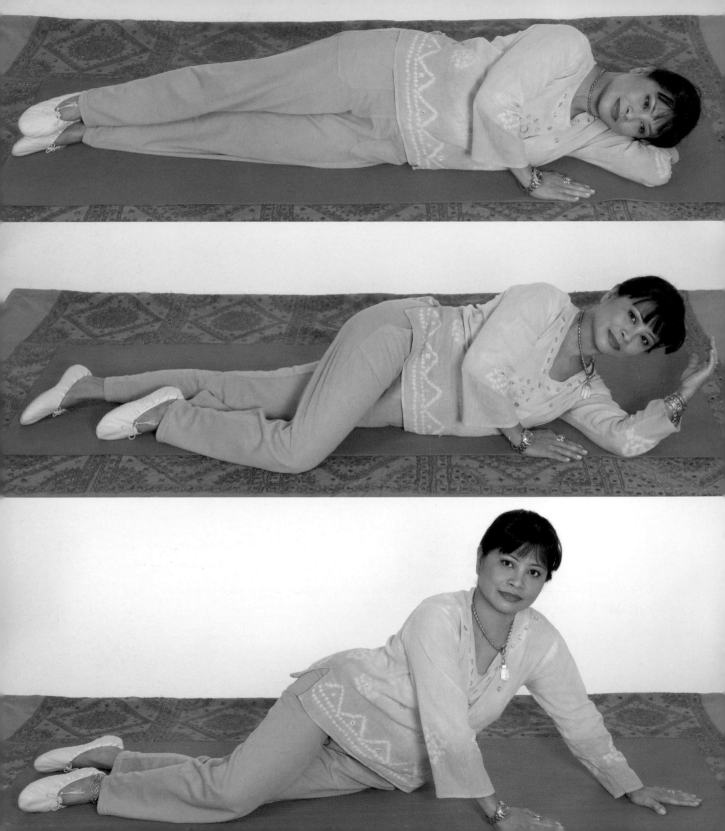

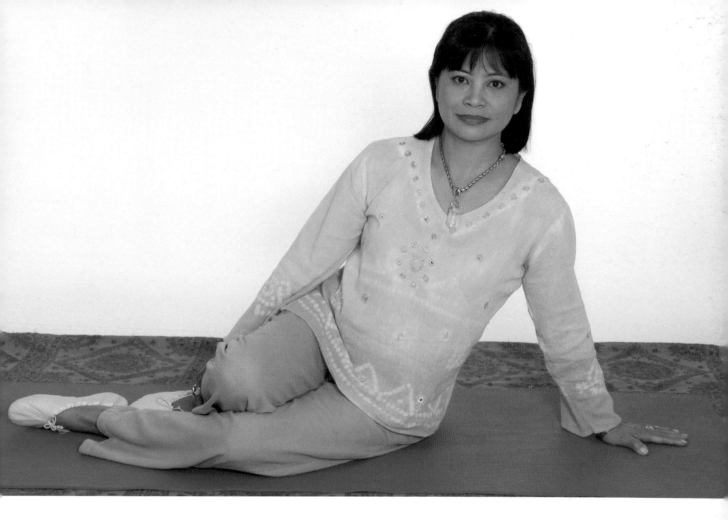

This concludes the abdominal excrcises. Give yourself plenty of time to come up into a sitting position. Get up from either the right or the left side by leaning on your free arm, straightening your back without straining it. Bend your knecs, and using your hands for support, slowly sit up straight.

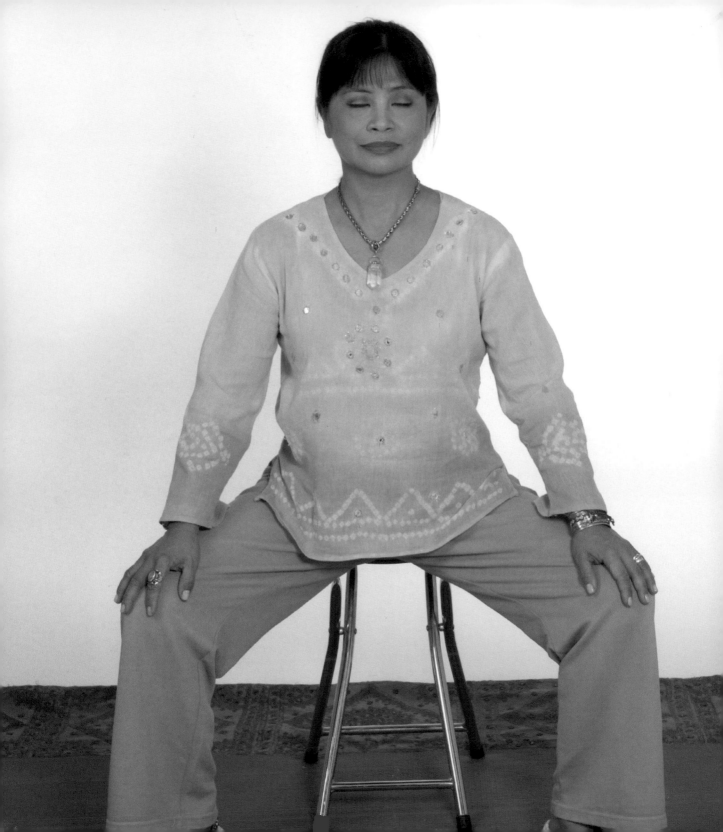

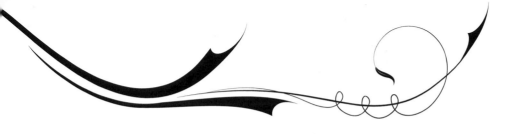

Spine Exercises

One does not encounter
"problems" but rather "situations"
in which one's capacity and
endurance are challenged.

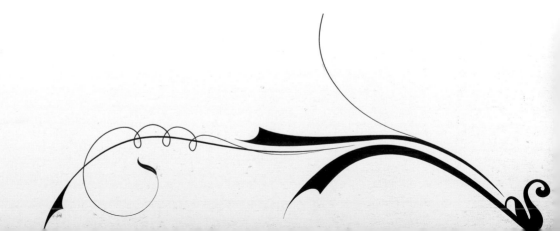

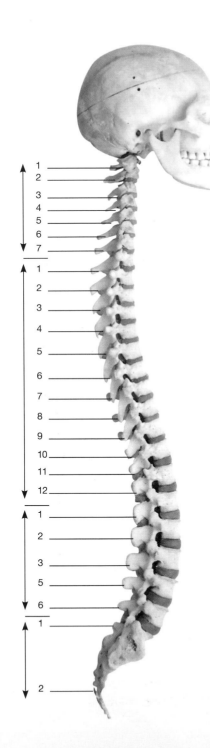

Illnesses Resulting from Calcification of the Cervical Spine

1st vertebra: headaches, nervousness, insomnia, migraines, epilepsy, high blood pressure, fatigue, and dizziness

2nd vertebra: sinus infections, allergies, deafness, vision problems, earaches, fainting, and in some cases blindness

3rd vertebra: face and arm pain (neuralgia) and skin blemishes

4th vertebra: hay fever and coughing

5th vertebra: laryngitis, sore throat, chronically runny nose, and angina

6th vertebra: backaches, arm pain, and tonsil inflammation

7th vertebra: colds and thyroid malfunction

Illnesses Resulting from Calcification of the Upper Spinal Column

1st vertebra: asthma, coughing, difficulty breathing, and arm and leg pain

2nd vertebra: arrhythmia and chest pain

3rd vertebra: bronchitis and pneumonia

4th vertebra: gallbladder malfunction and jaundice

5th vertebra: liver malfunction, anemia, circulation problems, and low blood pressure

6th vertebra: stomach problems and digestive problems

7th vertebra: diabetes, stomach ulcers, and gastritis

8th vertebra: anemia and hiccups

9th vertebra: allergies

10th vertebra: kidney malfunction, arteriosclerosis, exhaustion, and kidney infections

11th vertebra: skin irritation, pimples, and wrinkles

12th vertebra: bloating and infrequently sterility

Illnesses Resulting from Calcification of the Lower Spinal Column

1st vertebra: constipation and colitis

2nd vertebra: appendicitis, cramps, and varicose veins

3rd vertebra: bladder problems, menstruation discomfort, early menopause, impotence, incontinence, and knee pain

4th vertebra: sciatica, lumbago, and frequent urge to urinate

5th vertebra: poor leg circulation, cold feet, and "tired legs"

Discomfort Resulting from Calcification of the Sacrum

1st vertebra: sacroiliac pain

2nd vertebra: hemorrhoids, anal pruritus, and pain on the left side of the large intestine

Relaxing Your Spinal Column

Like the intestine, the spinal column—the body's third major organ—mirrors many different areas of our body according to the yoga practice. Health problems in the spine can also affect other organs, and thus they influence our body as a whole. The illustration at left shows examples of illnesses that can be brought about by either the calcification of the spine or an abnormality in the spine.

Spinal injuries, in particular, can lead to serious illness. For instance, impairment of 1st to 7th vertebrae in the cervical spine can cause problems in the eyes, neck, lungs, heart, throat, teeth, nose, and ears.

If you suffer from lung problems, the cause might be in the 2nd, 3rd, or the 4th vertebrae of the upper spinal column. Problems in the upper and lower vertebrae (T1–L3) can also cause illnesses of the bladder, appendix, prostate, and uterus, and may lead to impotence.

In order to make sure your spinal column remains healthy, you should do appropriate strengthening exercises on a regular basis. I will introduce these exercises in the following chapter. The illustrations will help make them clearer. If you do these exercises regularly, you will soon be free of neck, back, and lower-back pain.

Moreover, you will notice that your skin is clearer and your overall sense of well-being has improved.

Note: *If you have neck, upper-back, or lower-back problems, or suffer from hypertension, gastritis, or gastroesophageal reflux disease, please consult with your physician before doing these exercises.*

Neck (Cervical)

- ⇥ Sit on a chair with your legs spread apart.

- ⇥ Prop your elbows up on your knees and interlace your fingers.

- ⇥ Sit upright, and gently let your head fall forward to relax the neck muscles.

- ⇥ In this position, take 3 deep breaths in and out.

- ⇥ Take a deep breath; as you breathe out, turn your head to the right without lifting it up.

- ⇥ In this position, take 3 deep breaths in and out.

- ⇥ Take another deep breath; as you breathe out, turn your head to the middle. In this position, take 1 deep breath in and out.

- ⇥ Take another deep breath; as you breathe out, turn your head to the left without lifting it up.

- ⇥ In this position, take 3 deep breaths in and out.

- ⇥ Take another deep breath and turn your head to the middle as you breathe out. In this position, take 1 deep breath in and out.

Note: *If you have neck problems, please consult your doctor before doing this exercise.*

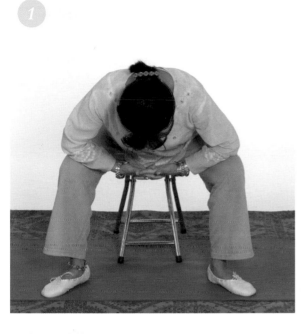

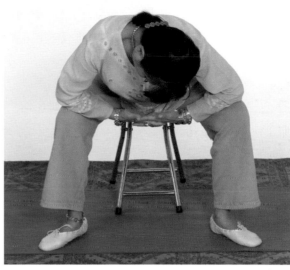

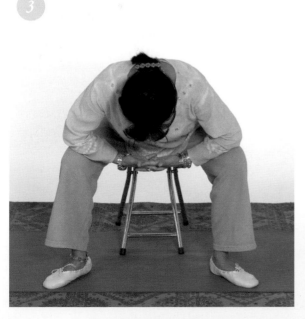

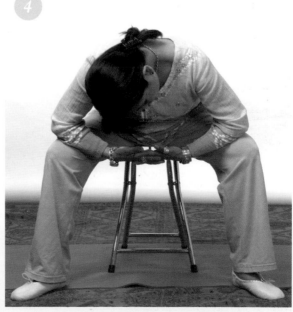

Back (Thoracic)

- Prop your elbows up on your knees and put your clasped hands in front of your chest. Lean your chest forward to your knees, as close to the thighs as you can. (If possible, rest your chest on your thighs.)

- Straighten your spine and gently drop your head forward. Make sure your shoulders stay down, your back is straight, and you are not bending too far forward.

- In this position, take 3 deep breaths in and out.

- Take another deep breath; as you breathe out, turn your head to the right without lifting it up.

- In this position, take 3 deep breaths in and out.

- Take another deep breath; as you breathe out, turn your head to the middle. In this position, take 1 deep breath in and out.

- Take another deep breath; as you breathe out, turn your head to the left without lifting it up.

- In this position, take 3 deep breaths in and out.

- Take another deep breath and turn your head to the middle as you breathe out. In this position, take 1 deep breath in and out.

Note: *If you have neck and lumbar spine problems, please consult your doctor before doing this exercise.*

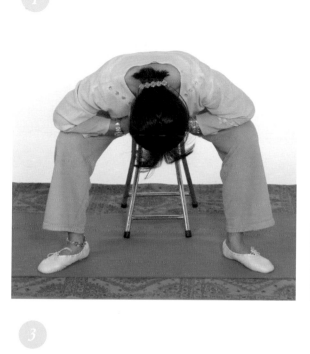

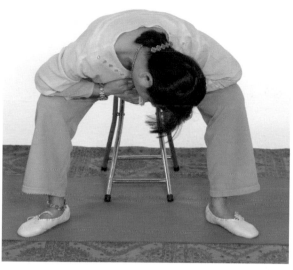

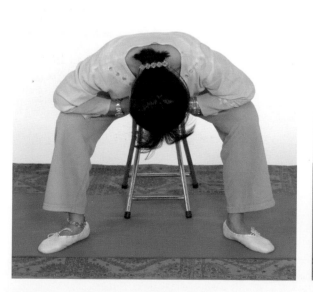

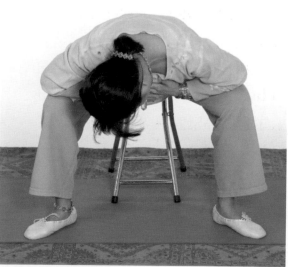

Spine Exercise 3

Pelvis (Lumbar)

- Sit on a chair with your legs spread apart. Keep yourself straight.

- Prop your elbows on your knees and let your upper body fold forward. Be careful not to strain your lower back, and make sure to keep your spine as straight as you can.

- Let your arms hang down, then cross them, holding onto your elbows.

- Let your head, neck, and shoulders hang loosely.

- Take a deep breath; as you breathe out, turn your upper body, at the waist, to the right. Your right elbow should touch your right calf.

- In this position, take 3 deep breaths in and out.

- Take another deep breath; as you breathe out, bring your arms and upper body back to the middle.

- In this position, take 1 deep breath in and out.

- Take another deep breath; as you breathe out, turn your upper body, at the waist, to the left. Your left elbow should touch your left calf.

- In this position, take 3 deep breaths in and out.

Note: *If you have high blood pressure, back and neck problems, gastritis, or acid reflux disease please consult your doctor before doing this exercise.*

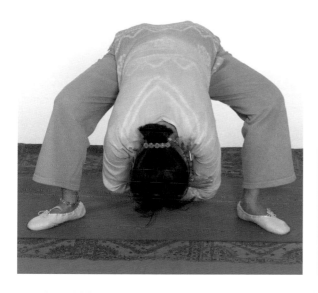

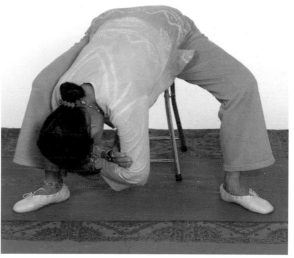

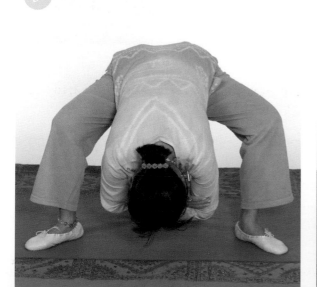

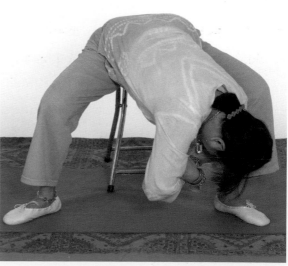

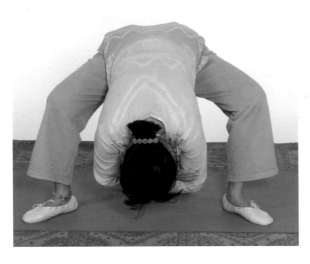

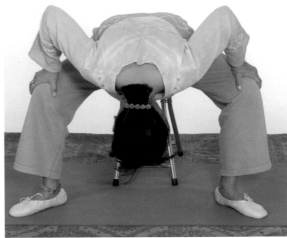

Straightening Up

꘎ Take another deep breath; as you breathe out, bring your arms and upper body back to the middle.

꘎ Prop your hands on your knees for support. Take a deep breath and slowly straighten the spine, pushing your hands against your knees for support. First straighten your lower back, then your belly area, then your chest and neck. Feel your arms stretch out. Stretch your neck and head toward the ceiling. Take a deep breath, hold it for about 5 seconds, and then release the tension and breathe out.

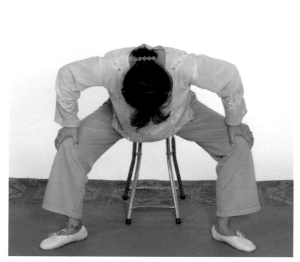

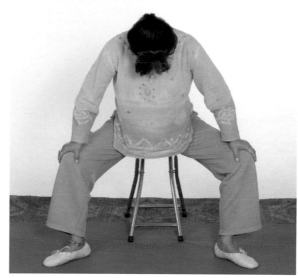

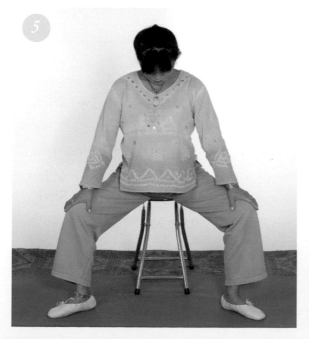

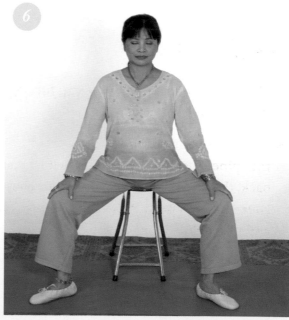

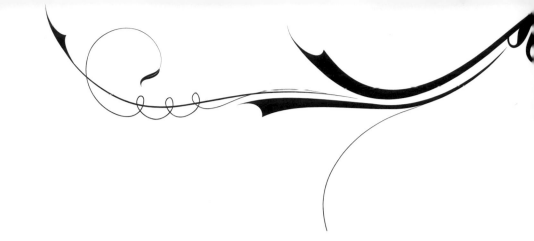

Woman is not just a lover;
She is the true light that shines
As though it had not been created,
She is its creator.

Mevlana Jalal-ud-din Rumi
Persian poet and Sufi master, 1207–1273

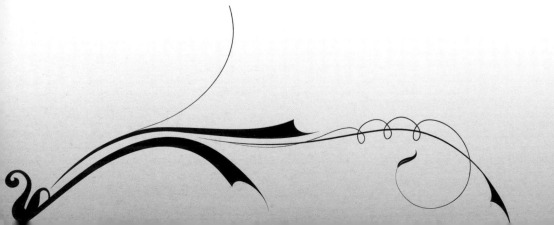

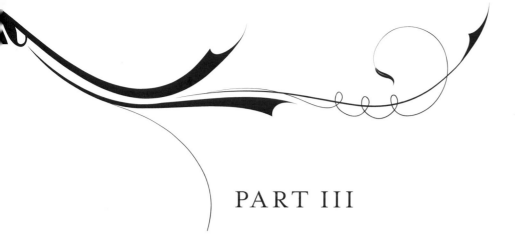

PART III

A Simple Daily Program

- ✦ Practice these yogic breathing exercises every morning. You can also repeat them over the course of the day while sitting or standing, whenever you have some extra time.

- ✦ Drink at least 1½ quarts of water a day.

- ✦ Eat plenty of raw fruits and vegetables.

- ✦ Practice the recommended face and body yoga exercises.

- ✦ Practice the face yoga exercises you have chosen at least 6 days a week.

- ✦ Do not do any face yoga exercises on the 7th day, so that your face can relax.

- ✦ Instead, you can continue doing the breathing exercises on the 7th day, along with the body exercises, making gentle, flowing movements.

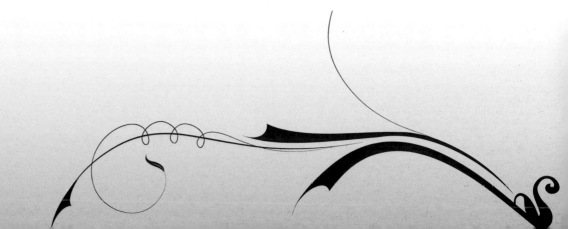

Basic Yoga Exercises
for a Radiant Presence

The body and face exercises can slow down your body's natural aging process and help you look up to ten years younger if you do them every day. The exercises for proper breathing, intestinal function, and spinal strength will also help give you a healthy, attractive, and vital appearance. At the same time, these exercises are important for your overall physical well-being.

Using Exercises and Relaxation for a Younger Appearance

Who doesn't want a radiant appearance and a healthy body? We know, of course, that we feel beautiful when our bodies look good. On the following pages, I provide you with a basic program to help build a beautiful, well-formed body in a short amount of time—as long as you do the exercises regularly.

Before we start this series of exercises, let us once again remember the meaning of "proper relaxation," one of the five principles of yoga:

Through proper relaxation, which creates calmness in body, mind, and spirit, we can correct and/or prevent stress-related pain and negative attitudes. Even at times when we cannot do the physical exercises, we can use relaxation techniques to strengthen our sense of well-being, achieve a positive attitude, and feel happy and young all over again.

TENSED	**RELAXED**

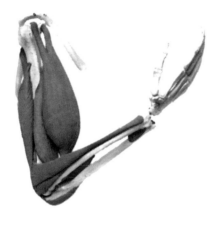

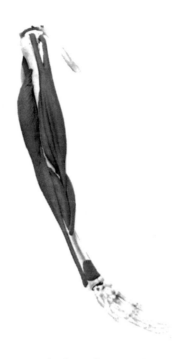

A tensed muscle. Long periods of tension without enough oxygen tire out muscles.

Muscles in a relaxed state. Muscles atrophy if they are not used.

Relaxation of Muscles

Proper relaxation is one of the five principles of yoga. In order to use it, you should first understand how our muscles work.

Our musculature uses more energy when in a contracted state (i.e., when getting ready for a movement; that is, while holding a "waiting" position) than it does in performing the actual movement. This creates tension and keeps the muscles from relaxing. However, if you can consciously relax your muscles during this phase, you will notice that they work more efficiently.

Kangaroo (Samakonasana)

Note: This exercise is intended for women who want to strengthen their pectoral muscles.

- Stand with your feet shoulder-width apart.
- Lean forward at a right angle, keeping your legs and back straight.
- Clasp your hands together.
- Take a deep breath; as you breathe out, firmly press your palms together. Hold for 5 seconds.
- Repeat this exercise at least 7 times.

Note: *If you have lower-back pain, you should do this position while sitting in a chair and should just make a slight forward bend. Make sure to keep your spine straight.*

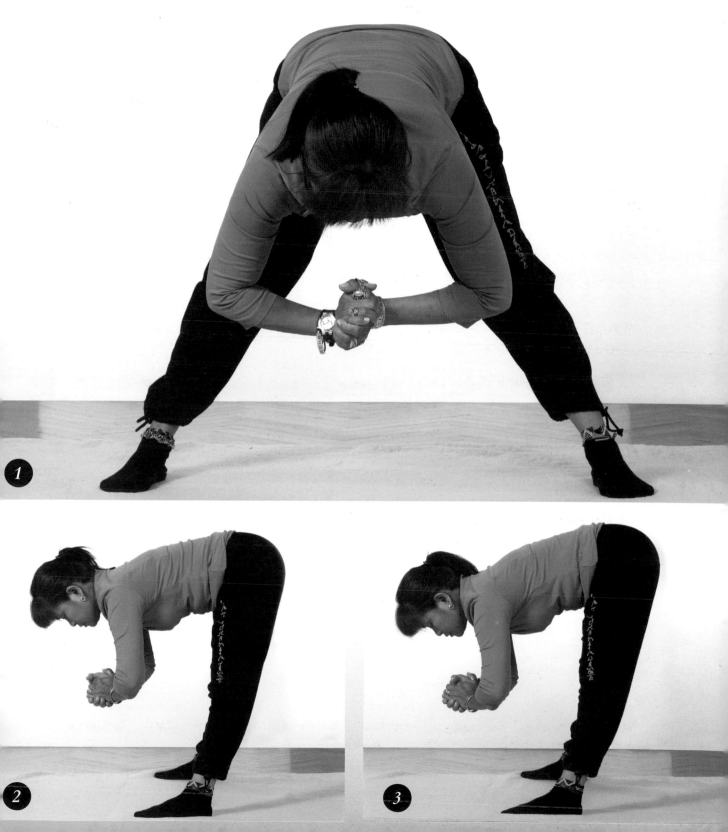

Cat/Tiger Pose (Vyaghrasana I)

Strengthens the spine, chest, and internal organs

- Kneel on all fours. Make sure that your hands and knees are shoulder-width apart.
- Breathe in and lift your head up toward the nape of your neck. Sink your abdomen toward the floor, but keep your pelvis high.
- As you breathe out, draw your chin in toward your chest; pull in your belly, hold it tight, and arch your back like a cat.
- Repeat this exercise 7 times.

Note: *If you have minor knee problems, use a soft blanket and make sure your knees are in a comfortable position. If you have major knee problems, do this exercise sitting on a chair and just try to flex your spine gently forward and backward.*

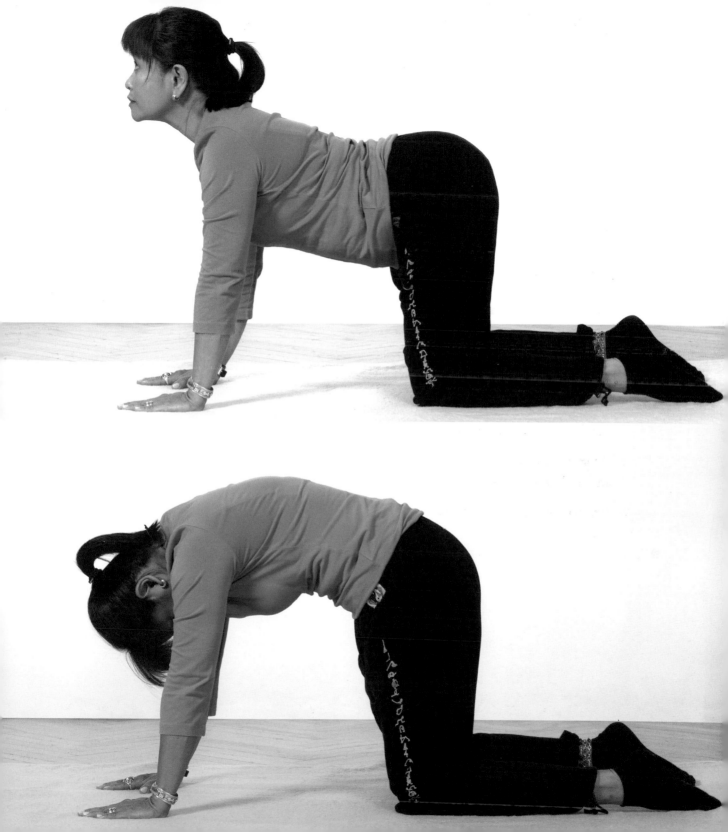

Horse Kick (Vyaghrasana II)

Shapes hips and legs

- Kneel on all fours, keeping your back straight and your hands and knees shoulder-width apart.

- Breathe in and bring your right knee up to your chin. As you breathe out, stretch your right leg out behind you and toward the ceiling as far as you can. Keep your toes pointed, and hold the breath and the position for a count of 7.

- Repeat this exercise 7 times, and then do the same sequence with the left leg.

Note: *If you have major knee problems, please do not do this exercise. If you have minor knee problems, check with your physician beforehand. Use a soft blanket and make sure your knees are in a comfortable position.*

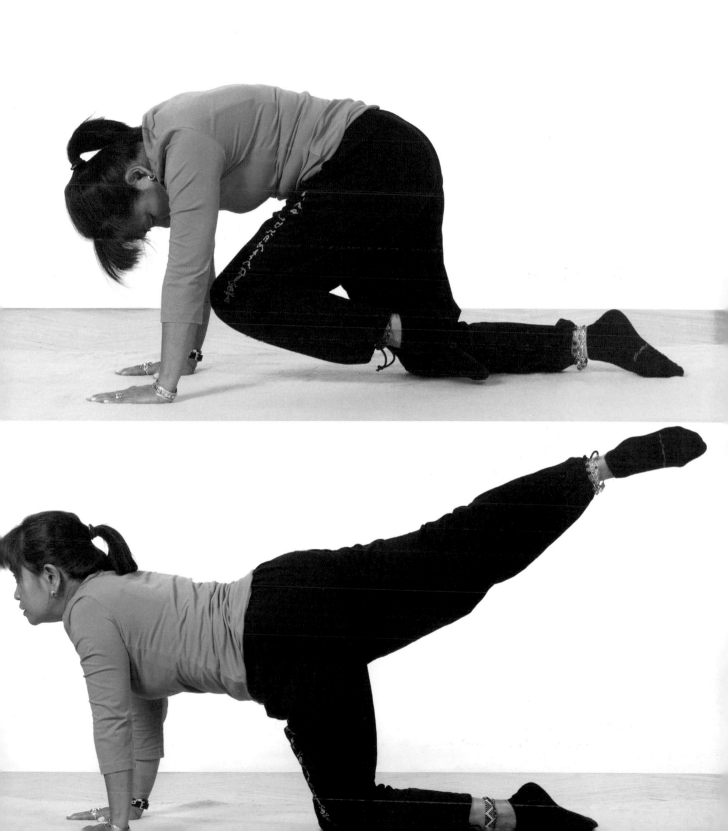

Dog Pose (Vygahrasana III)

Shapes hips and legs

- Kneel on all fours.
- Breathe in. Lift your right leg with the knee bent, and reach it out to the side like a dog marking its territory.
- Now stretch out your right leg until it is parallel to the floor, point your toes, and hold the position for about 7 seconds.
- As you breathe out, bend your leg and return to the starting position.
- Repeat the exercise 7 times on each side, alternating sides.

Note: *If you have major knee problems, please do not do this exercise. If you have minor knee problems, check with your physician beforehand. Use a soft blanket and make sure your knees are in a comfortable position.*

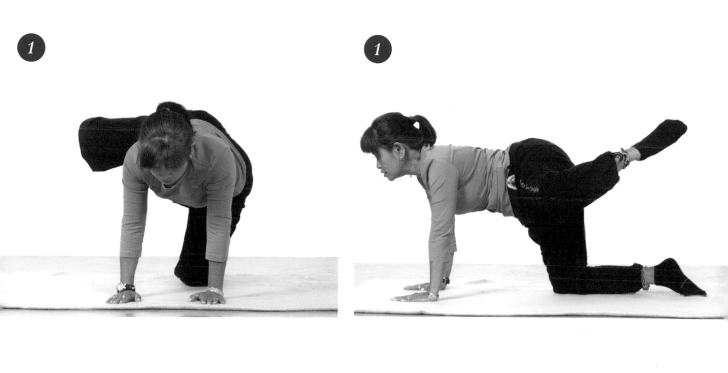

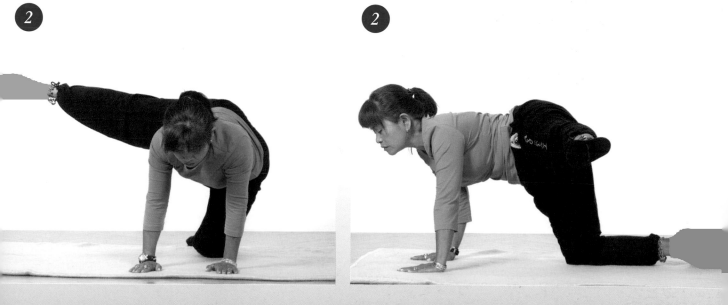

Baby Walk

For a trim waistline

This exercise has a natural massaging effect on the spine and on all the internal organs. It also promotes circulation and digestion, and reduces sciatic pain.

- Sit on the floor with your legs straight out in front of you. Cross your arms in front of your chest. With your pelvis and legs on the floor, take 7 small "wiggling steps" forward and then back, without bending the knees. (Try to walk with your buttocks and just slide your legs as you move backward or forward.)

- As you move forward with your right hip and the right side of your pelvis, turn your upper body to the left. Then do the same thing on the other side, turning your upper body to the right.

- Repeat this exercise 7 times going forward and 7 times going backward.

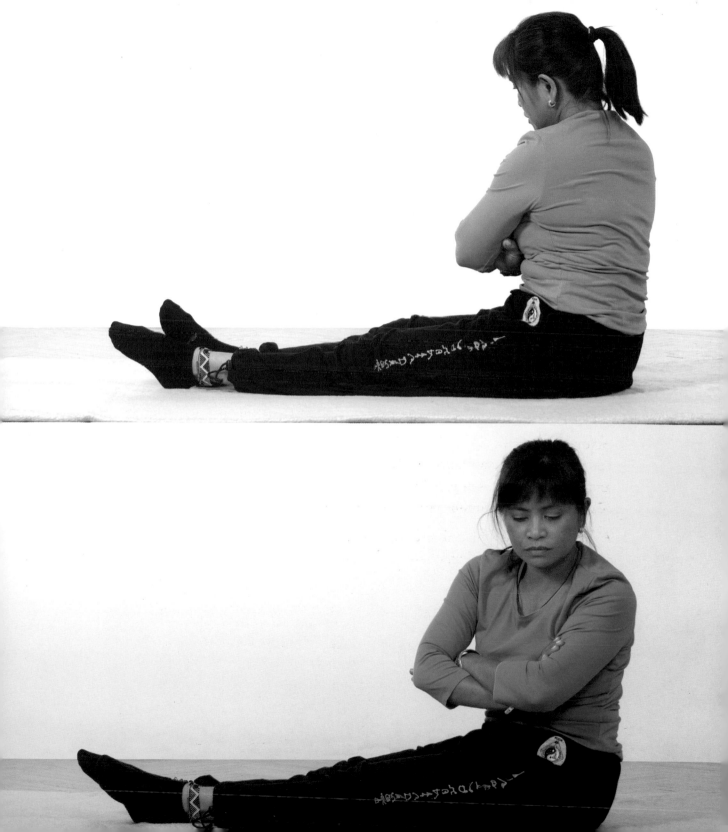

Half Bridge (Ardha Sethubandhasana)

For the bladder, reproductive organs, and large intestine

- Lie on the floor and bend your knees, with your feet shoulder-width apart.

- Hold on to your ankles with your hands.

- Take a deep breath and push your pelvis as far upward as you can, contracting the pelvic and anal muscles.

- Tighten your belly and gluteal muscles, and hold your breath and this position for a count of 7.

- As you breathe out, bring your pelvis back to the starting position. Repeat this exercise 7 times.

- When you bring your pelvis upward for the 8th time, hold this position and take 20 short bellows breaths from the belly.

- Then go into the Relaxation Pose (see pages 114–115).

Note: *If you have high stomach acidity or acid reflux, do not exert yourself too much while doing these exercises. The exercises should also not be done during menstruation or on a full stomach.*

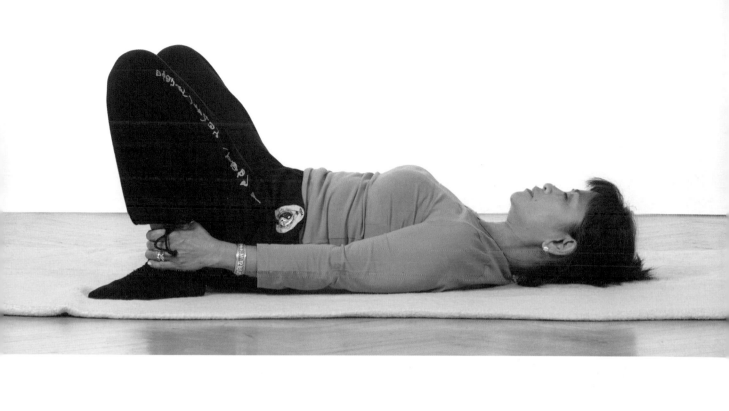

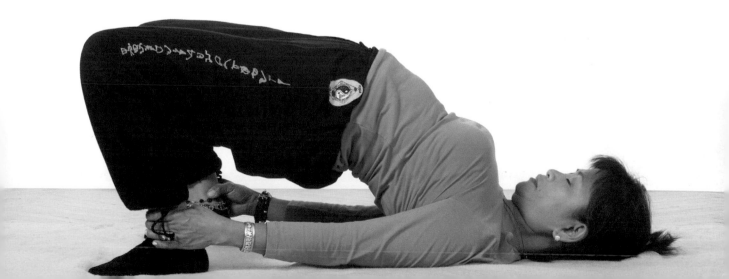

7

Flapping Butterfly

Strengthens and tones the upper arms

- Stand up with a straight spine. Let your arms hang to the sides of your body. Then draw your arms slightly backward, pushing your rib cage forward.
- Your palms should be facing forward with your fingers together.
- Now flap your arms sideways like a bird at least 100 times.

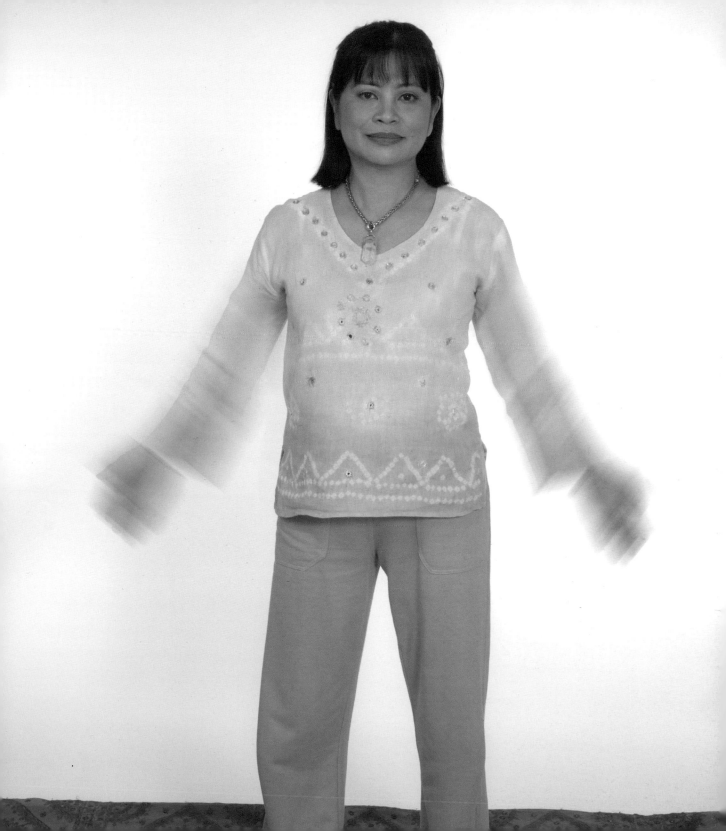

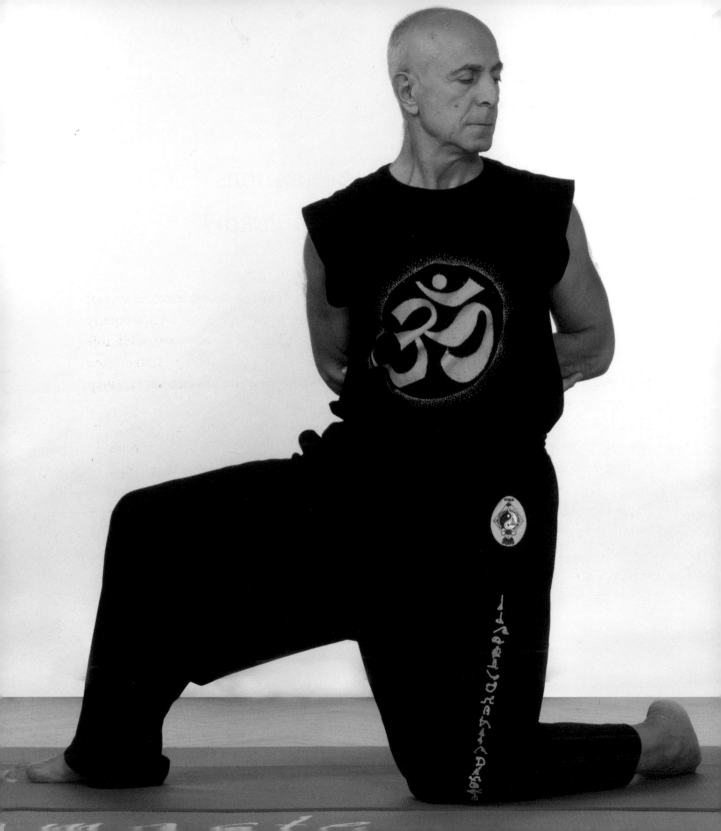

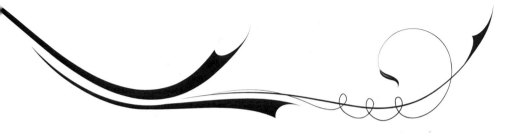

Sun and Moon Salutations (Surya–Chandra Namaskar)

The Sun and Moon Salutations are exercise sequences that have been used in Asia for several centuries to promote good health. The sun and the moon are considered to be life-energy sources. While the sun represents masculine energy, or yang, the moon represents the feminine, or yin. This exercise, which you can do in the morning and the evening, balances the positive yang and negative yin energies in your body. Doing this series of exercises can help you become healthier and more vital, content, and balanced.

Try to do the 30-exercise sequence without strain, fluidly and elegantly, and while maintaining proper breathing. In order to complete a sequence, you should do all 30 exercises in a row. Depending on your physical condition, you can also repeat the sequence a couple of times.

These exercises activate more than one hundred muscles in your body. This makes your body much more flexible, since every body part is being used. The exercises will help balance your body and its energy flow. If you do the Sun and Moon Salutations daily while following the basic rules for good health, you will have a livelier, more-energetic, smoother, and more-flexible body.

Note: If you have minor knee problems, use a thick blanket to help support them.

1. Prayer Pose (Pranamasana)
Stand upright with your feet nearly touching. Fold your hands in front of your rib cage. With your eyes closed, take 3 deep breaths.

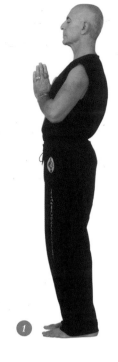

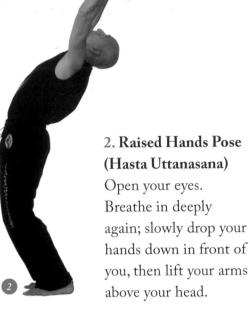

2. Raised Hands Pose (Hasta Uttanasana)
Open your eyes. Breathe in deeply again; slowly drop your hands down in front of you, then lift your arms above your head.

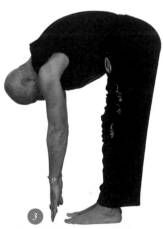

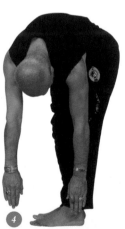

3. Feet to Hands Pose (Padahastasana) As you breathe out, bend your upper body forward and downward until your fingers or hands touch the floor. Breathe in and out 3 times in this position. (If you have back problems, bend your knees.)

4. Slowly swing from side to side with your arms dangling; breathe in as you swing to the right, and breathe out as you swing to the left.

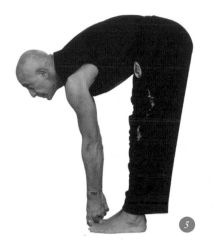

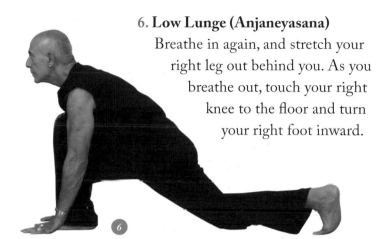

6. Low Lunge (Anjaneyasana)

Breathe in again, and stretch your right leg out behind you. As you breathe out, touch your right knee to the floor and turn your right foot inward.

5. Take another deep breath and touch your toes. (If you are unable to do this or if you have lower-back problems, bend your knees.) Look straight ahead and press your tongue to the roof of your mouth. Take 3 deep breaths in and out in this position.

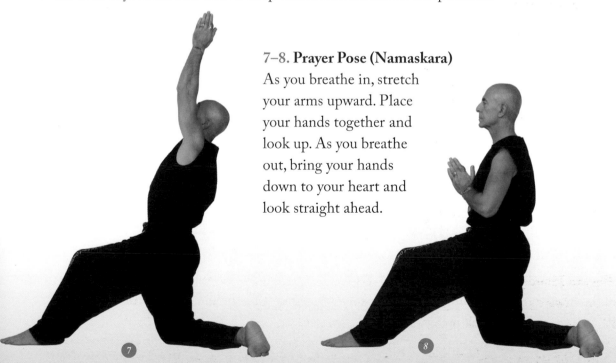

7–8. Prayer Pose (Namaskara)

As you breathe in, stretch your arms upward. Place your hands together and look up. As you breathe out, bring your hands down to your heart and look straight ahead.

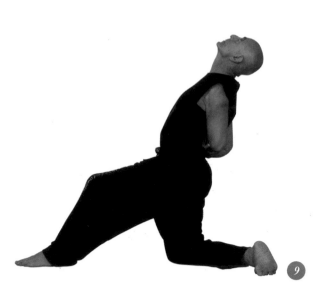

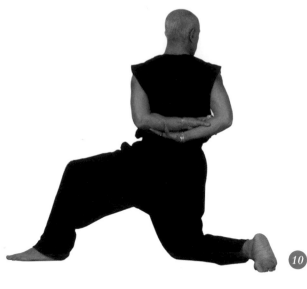

9. Camel Pose variation (Ustrasana)
Breathe in; cross your arms behind your back. Lean back a little, and look upward as you breathe out. Take another breath, and straighten your upper body (i.e., bring it back to the middle) as you breathe out.

10. Breathe in; as you breathe out, turn your upper body to the right and look behind you. Take another breath, and straighten your upper body as you breathe out.

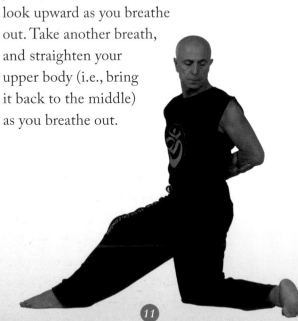

11. Breathe in; as you breathe out, turn your upper body to the left and look behind you. Take another breath, and straighten your upper body as you breathe out.

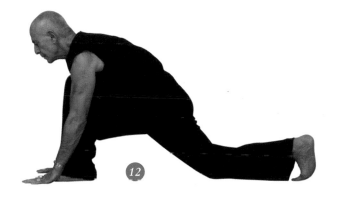

12. Low Lunge (Anjaneyasana)
Breathe in; as you breathe out, place your hands on the floor on either side of your left foot.

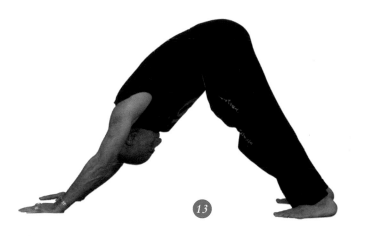

13. Mountain Pose (Parvatasana)
Breathe in, and stretch your left leg out behind you, putting both feet beside each other. As you breathe out, lower your head between your arms and press both heels toward the floor. (Some traditions also call this well-known pose "Downward-Facing Dog.")

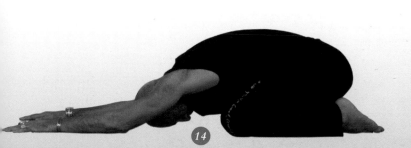

14. Hare Pose (Shashankasana)
Breathe in; as you breathe out, bend your knees. Kneel on the floor with your knees shoulder-width apart, then lower your upper body forward. Stretch out your arms and touch your forehead to the floor. Take 3 deep breaths in and out in this position.

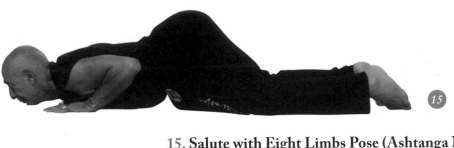

15. Salute with Eight Limbs Pose (Ashtanga Namaskara)
Take another breath; as you breathe out, slide yourself forward like a snake, keeping your knees, hands, chest, and chin on the floor.

16. Cobra Pose (Bhujangasana) Breathe in, lift your head and your upper body. Your arms should be straight and your shoulders down. Hold this pose and take 3 deep breaths in and out.

> *Note: If you have lower-back pain or problems, keep your forearms and elbows on the floor, bend your upper body only slightly, and take 3 deep breaths in and out.*

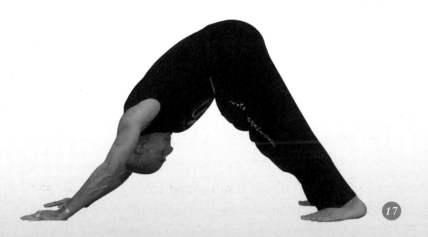

17. Mountain Pose (Parvatasana) Take another breath, place your feet on the floor, and as you breathe out, raise your pelvis upward, letting your head hang down loosely between your arms. Take 3 deep breaths in and out in this position.

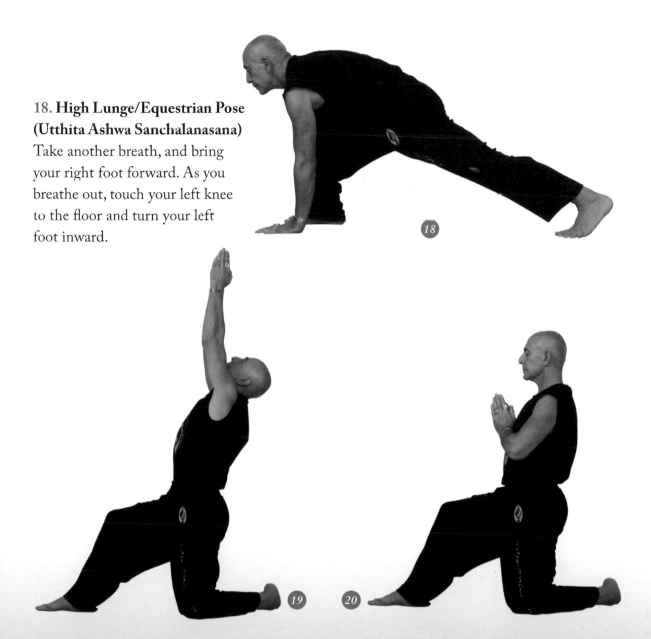

18. High Lunge/Equestrian Pose (Utthita Ashwa Sanchalanasana) Take another breath, and bring your right foot forward. As you breathe out, touch your left knee to the floor and turn your left foot inward.

19–20. Prayer Pose (Namaskara) Breathe in, and stretch your arms upward. Place your hands together, and then look up. As you breathe out, bring your hands down to your heart while looking straight ahead.

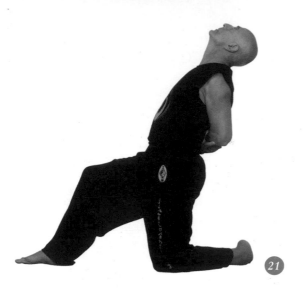

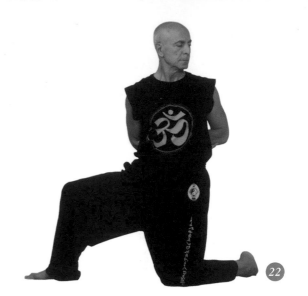

21. Camel Pose (Ustrasana) Breathe in; cross your arms behind your back. Lean back a little and look upward as you breathe out. Take another breath, and straighten your upper body as you breathe out.

22. Breathe in; as you breathe out, turn your upper body to the left and look over your shoulder. Take another breath, and straighten your upper body as you breathe out.

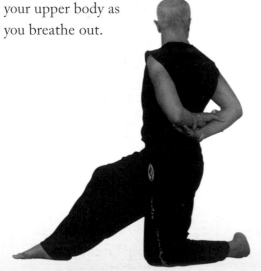

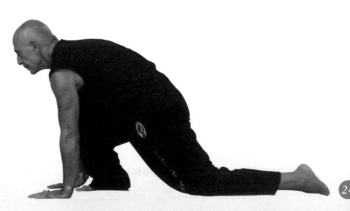

23. Breathe in; as you breathe out, turn your upper body to the right and look over your shoulder. Take another breath, and straighten your upper body as you breathe out.

24. Breathe in; as you breathe out, place your hands on the floor on either side of your right foot. Take another breath; bring your left foot forward and place it next to your right foot.

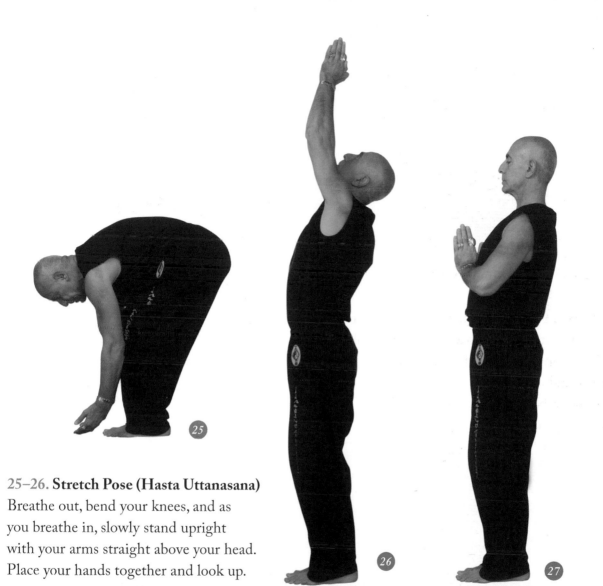

25–26. Stretch Pose (Hasta Uttanasana)
Breathe out, bend your knees, and as
you breathe in, slowly stand upright
with your arms straight above your head.
Place your hands together and look up.

27. Prayer Pose (Pranamasana) As you breathe out, bring your hands down to your heart and
hold them in front of your rib cage in the "namasté" position. Take one last deep breath in, and
let it out.

Do this series one more time, but use your left leg in steps 6 and 18. Together, this makes up
one sequence. I recommend doing the Sun and Moon Salutations 3 times.

Relaxation Pose (Shavasana)

- Lie on the floor and close your eyes.
- Your legs should be shoulder-width apart.
- Your arms should be 8–12 inches away from your body.
- Have your palms facing up and your hands relaxed.
- Relax your entire body and take 6 deep breaths in and out.
- With every breath, you will feel yourself growing more and more relaxed.
- Breathe normally. Banish all thoughts. Think about nothing.
- In order to "control" your mind, imagine that you are able to look at your third eye. Try to concentrate on only your breathing.
- Stay in this position for at least 5 minutes. Then slowly sit upright and prepare yourself for the meditation.

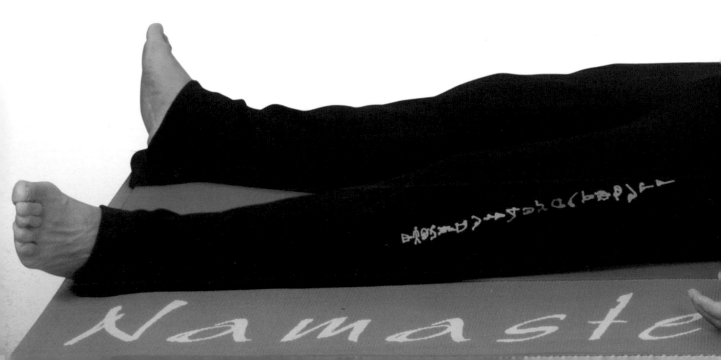

Why This Exercise Is Useful

- The Relaxation Pose is relaxing and builds up your energy. It keeps your body, soul, and mind in harmony.

- It frees you from tension, creates vitality, and increases your awareness.

- It strengthens your circulation, regulates your blood pressure, calms your mind and soul, and prevents stress. The exercise is also considered a preliminary stage to meditation. It helps you direct your attention inward, and it has a therapeutic effect on physical and mental ailments.

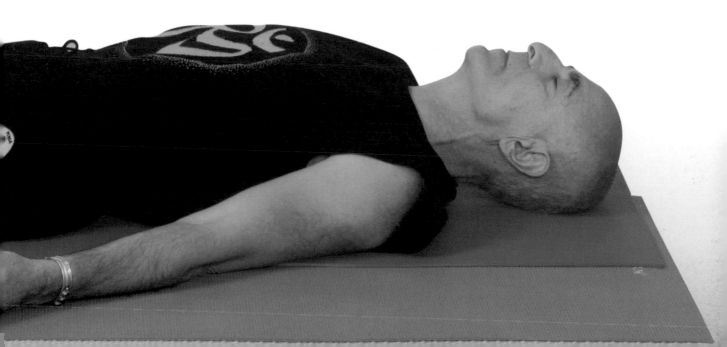

Breathing Before Meditation (Pranayam)

Look in the chapter entitled "The Power of Hand Gestures: Mudras" (page 119) and choose a mudra for the pranayam breathing exercise before starting the meditation.

- Before starting the exercise, breathe out.
- Close your eyes and silently count to 4 as you breathe in.
- Hold your breath and silently count to 4.
- Breathe out, silently counting to 4.
- Hold your breath, silently counting to 4.
- Repeat this meditation breathing exercise at least 7 times.

The Meditation

- Place your hands in the first position of the mudra for this meditation.
- Breathe normally, and imagine that you are breathing easily in and out.
- Relax with your eyes closed, and empty your mind. Don't think about anything, and don't wish for anything.
- In order to control your mind, with eyes closed, imagine that you are looking into the third eye between your eyebrows. Keep the awareness on your breath.
- Stay in this position for as long as you want, without moving.
- To end the meditation, take a deep breath, and as you slowly breathe out from your diaphragm, say, "om," in a natural and soft voice. Breathe in again.
- As you breathe out, run the palms of your hands across your eyes, moving outward.
- Do a brief facial stretch by squinting, frowning, smiling, opening and closing the mouth and eyes, and squeezing in every direction.
- Take a deep breath, and using both hands rub your whole face upward in one direction from the chin, to the forehead, and all the way to the back of the head and to the nape of the neck.
- Fold your hands in front of your rib cage, lower your head a little, and end the meditation.
- Namaste!

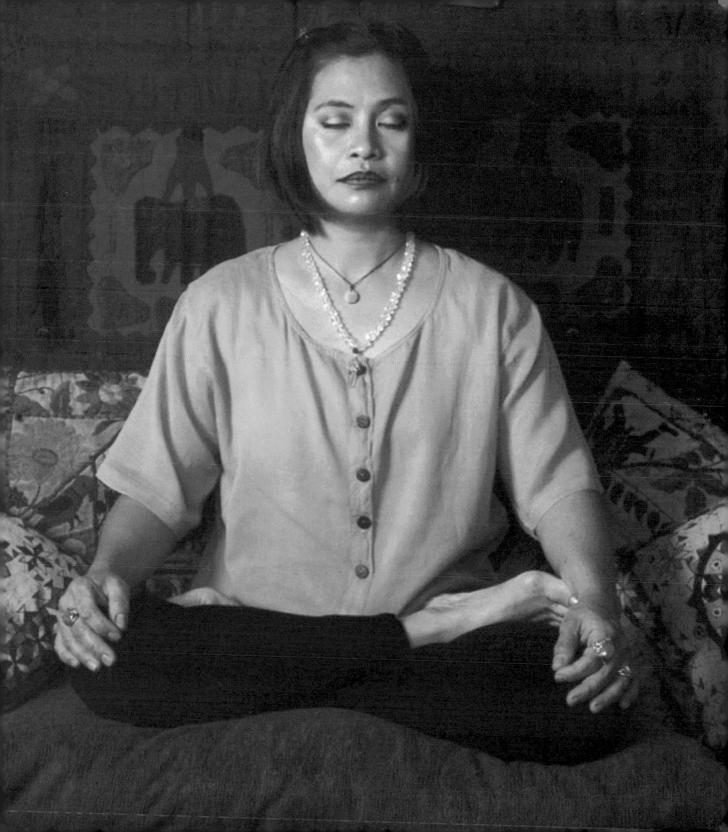

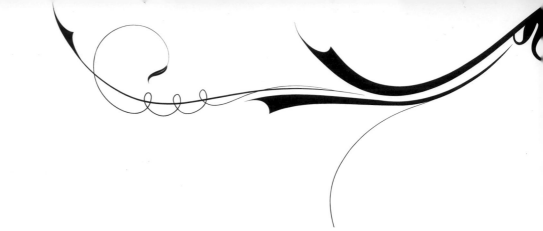

There is an invisible being. Do not think you are alone!
He has very sensitive and sharp ears.
Avoid saying bad things.

Mevlana Jalal-ud-din Rumi

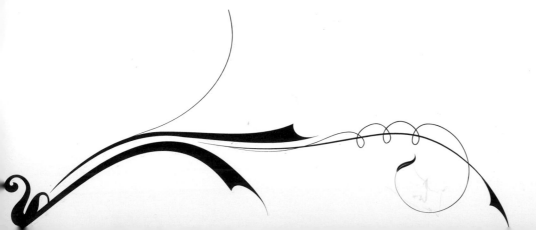

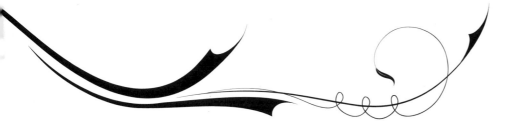

The Power of Hand Gestures: Mudras

In traditional yoga, breathing exercises and meditation are accompanied by specific hand positions or gestures. These positions are called hand mudras. They represent the basic elements of life—such as earth, fire, air, space, and water—and they are meant to activate the healing power of nature and strengthen the immune system.

The basic elements are associated with the following fingers:

Thumb: fire/sun
Index finger: air/breath
Middle finger: sky/space
Ring finger: earth/body
Pinky finger: water/energy

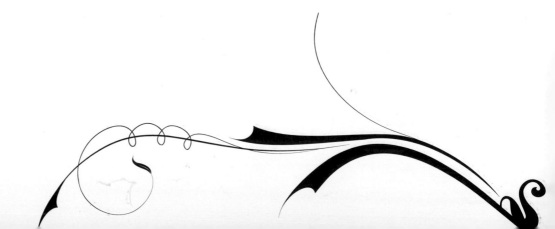

Meditation Mudra

The tips of the thumb and index finger
touch very gently.

What this position does:
It strengthens brain activity,
concentration, and memory.
It also helps prevent insomnia, tension,
and lack of concentration, and it
supports meditation.

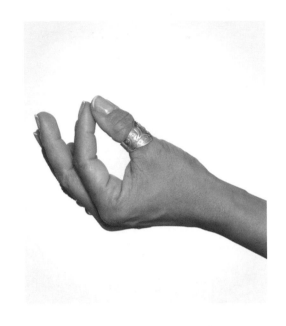

Energy Mudra

The thumb is placed in the palm of the hand,
and the other four fingers enclose the thumb.

What this position does:
It allows you to hold your breath longer,
promotes blood circulation, and increases
lung capacity. It strengthens the entire body.
You are able to take longer breaths, and
fewer of them. Indian philosophy does not
measure life in minutes, days, months, or
years, but by the number of breaths. Thus,
if you hold the "pure air" in your lungs long
enough, it is said to lengthen your life.

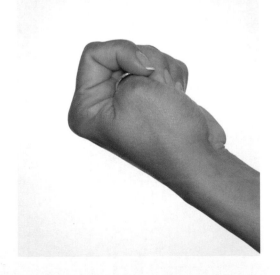

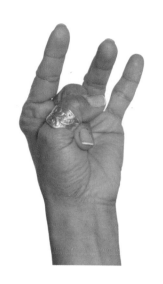

Shunya Mudra (Cosmic Energy)

Bend your middle finger down until it touches the base of the palm of your hand, then gently press the middle finger down using your thumb.

What this position does:
It helps heal earaches and works to prevent dizziness and general hearing problems. To maximize its effectiveness, you should hold this mudra position for 40 to 60 minutes.

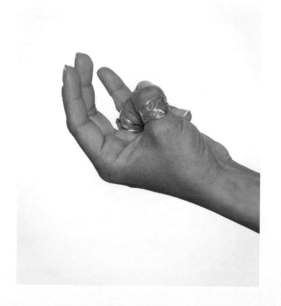

Sun Mudra

Bend your ring finger down, and press into the end of your ring finger with your thumb.

What this position does:
It raises body temperature, eases digestive problems, and helps the body break down fat.

Varun Mudra (Water Energy)

The tips of the thumb and pinky finger touch.

What this position does:
It helps purify the blood and heal skin irritations, and it improves overall skin condition. It also helps with stomach problems caused by dehydration.

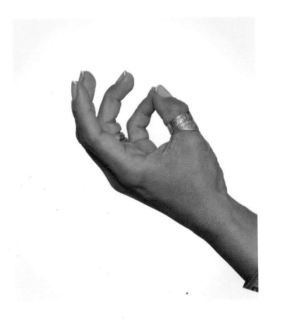

Pritvi Mudra (Earth and Body Energy)

Gently place the tips of your thumbs and ring fingers together.

What this position does:
It increases life energy, gives you strength to recover from illness, and creates peace of mind.

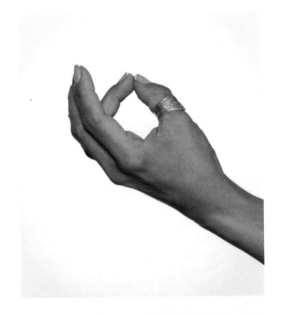

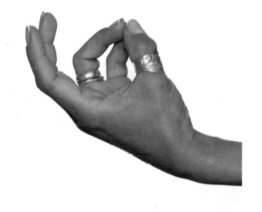

Prana Mudra (Life Energy)

The pinky and ring fingers touch. The tip of the thumb rests on the tips of these fingers, creating a connection.

What this position does:
It increases life energy and the body's vitality, along with inner balance, and relieves nervousness and fatigue. It also improves eyesight.

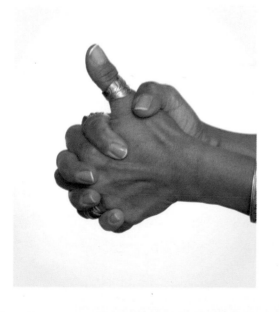

Ling Mudra

Fold your hands and straighten your left thumb, pointing it upward. Your right index finger and right thumb should enclose your left thumb.

What this position does:
It increases life energy and strengthens the respiratory system. It creates body heat that helps the body burn more fat, and it reduces mucus excretion. If you do this exercise, you should drink plenty of fluids.

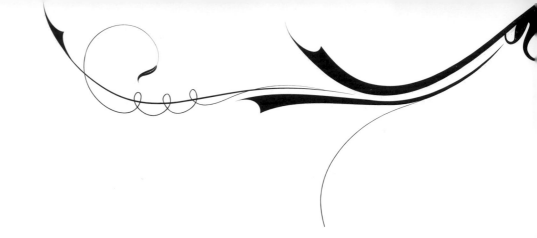

Give up straw and barley;
Start to eat basil and roses!
The physical belly leads to the barn
The spiritual belly leads to fields of basil.

Mevlana Jalal-ud-din Rumi

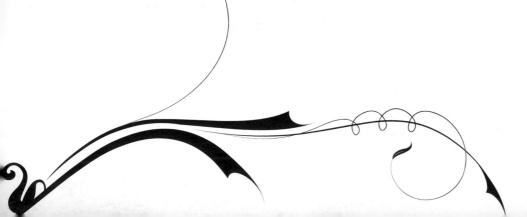

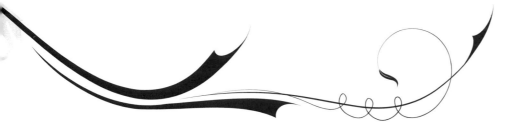

Good Nutrition

You have already learned that good nutrition is one of the five yogic principles. If you want to achieve good results in the short term by doing the face-yoga and the breathing, abdominal, and spine exercises, along with the body-toning exercises, I recommend that you also pay attention to proper nutrition. In this chapter I will describe proper nutrition according to the yogic principles.

The gift of food should not be used only for the sake of pleasure, just as sexuality is more than simple lust. You might imagine the lust in sexuality as a side effect of conception and birth. In the same way, we take in nutrients for the purpose of survival, and the pleasure we get from eating is a tempting bonus that encourages people to eat.

Unfortunately, humanity has lost its instinctive connection with nature. We are no longer able to determine what is good or bad for us.

Today, both Western and Eastern cultures carry out scientific studies to remind people how to live healthy lives and/or regain their good health. In this context, good nutrition means focusing on foods that are found in nature, such as fruit, vegetables, dried fruits, grains, herbs, and plants. These vital, nutrient-rich foods should be eaten raw or at least only half-cooked. This will give you a balanced diet and prevent many illnesses, allowing you to lead a healthier life.

Uncooked foods contain life energy, or prana. If vegetables are cooked too long, this energy is lost. Of course, you may not always be able to eat only raw foods. But you can choose to eat fewer foods that have been treated with hormones or other chemicals, along with sugar, white flour, starches, cooked foods, and meat. We have the ability to make changes, and eating well is one of the most important ways to lead a healthy life without illness.

The digestion process starts in the mouth. This means that proper, thorough chewing can help our bodies take in nutrients and process them more efficiently. The enzymes in saliva help digest starches and carbohydrates, so you should chew your food until it is mushy. Also, it is easier for your stomach muscles to assist in digestion if you stop eating before you feel full.

The best time to drink water or liquids in general is either half an hour before or 2 to 3 hours after eating. Eating too much protein, or too many different kinds of protein, during a meal will hinder your digestive process and cause your body to age more rapidly.

Your body absorbs the ingredients in food through the walls of the intestine. This is why it is important to cleanse the intestines of mucus and blockages; otherwise, the minerals and vitamins in your healthy diet cannot be fully absorbed through the intestinal walls, into the bloodstream and cells. You should eat only small amounts of meat, starchy foods, and dairy products, which are all sticky and produce mucus. For more on this topic, I recommend The Mucusless Diet Healing System by Professor Arnold Ehrets (1976).

People who spend too much time driving or sitting, or who don't get enough water, exercise, or proper nutrition tend to suffer from constipation. Constipation is a serious health risk. When constipated, the body does not eliminate waste and toxins on a regular basis, which causes illness. In order to prevent constipation, I recommend drinking eight to ten glasses of water between meals.

- Think positive!

- Only eat after your last meal has been properly digested and you feel hungry again.

- Share your food with people who have less.

- Cheese and ice cream are the most fattening foods.

- Burned oil is toxic; avoid fried foods.

- In order to be fully beneficial, fruit should be eaten an hour before mealtime, on an empty

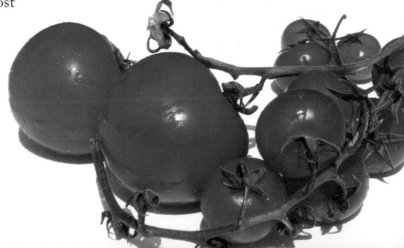

stomach. To avoid digestive discomfort when you are sleeping, do not eat fruit after meals or just before bedtime.

- Eat vegetables and salad with every meal.

- If you have to eat something unhealthy because there are no other options, eat it on an empty stomach and wait until it is completely digested before eating anything else.

- Only put as much on your plate as you can eat. Don't waste anything—remember that many people in the world are starving.

- After a day when you have eaten too much, spend one to two days consuming only water, vegetable juices, and fruit juices or vegetable soup and fruit. If you feel hungry, you can eat a salad or small servings of vegetables. Drink plenty of water.

- For 5 or 6 days a week, make sure you eat at the right time of day and have a good combination of foods. Take the other day or two "off." On those days, you can eat whatever you want, in moderation. This will not harm your body, and it will relieve stress.

- Fasting can be useful. I fast once a week with water. This allows my body to rest and eliminate toxins. While fasting, I don't drink too much water—1½ quarts at most—and I drink it a sip at a time. Sometimes fasting can cause headaches and dizziness, because our bodies are used to having food at certain times. Instead, our body draws on its food stores, but it also processes its stored toxins. This can lead to dizziness, headaches, and nausea. In order to prevent these reactions, it is a good idea to drink water to wash the toxins out of the body.

- There are many advantages to a vegetarian diet. However, geographic location and lifestyle play an important role in determining whether a vegetarian diet is right for you. For instance, people who were born and grew up in Alaska can regulate their body temperature by eating meat, and vegetables are not cultivated there. On the other hand, people who live in warm regions age faster and are subject to disease if they eat too much red meat.

⧎ Nowadays, fruit and vegetables are grown out of season in greenhouses and cows, sheep, goats, and chickens are bred and farmed in large assembly-line operations that are like factories. When these animals are slaughtered, their cells are filled with negative emotions such as sadness, anger, and stress; this releases harmful hormones that affect the quality of the meat we consume.

⧎ Each of us has a specific genetic predisposition. Thus, we are also predisposed for certain diseases, even if we feel healthy now. For example, if your grandfather, father, or mother has lung disease, you are also liable to develop this disease. In that case you should avoid everything that could negatively affect your lungs, such as cigarettes and alcohol.

⧎ Your diet can predict how you will age. If you eat too many carbohydrates and too much sugar, you will have a rougher complexion as you age, with more wrinkles and sagging skin.

⧎ In order to keep our acid-base metabolism in balance, we should eat up to 80 percent basic and 20 percent acidic foods. Excess acidity in the body is the cause of many illnesses. Minerals like sulfur, phosphorus, iodine, and chlorine create acids, while calcium, magnesium, potassium, sodium, and iron create bases.

⧎ It is important to pay attention to the foods we combine, because digesting different foods requires different enzymes, different acid levels, different mediums, and different digestion times. In the following pages you will find a list of healthy food combinations.

The ego is like
A band, a chain, and you are like
Prisoners who are chained to it.
Take up the pick to
Escape from the dungeon! When you
Break free from the dungeon, you shall become the sultan,
You shall be the commander.

Mevlana Jalal-ud-din Rumi

Healthy and Unhealthy Food Combinations

1. Perfect combinations of food

2. Acceptable combinations of food (at most 4 times a month)

3. Less preferable combinations of food (at most 2 times a month)

0. Nonrecommended combinations of food (at most once a month)

	Meat, chicken, fish	Legumes	Butter, cream
Meat, chicken, fish		2	0
Legumes	2		2
Butter, cream	0	2	
Yogurt	0	2	0
Plant oils	1	1	0
Sugar, sugary foods	0	0	0
Bread, potatoes, rice, noodles	3	3	2
Sour fruit, tomato paste	3	3	3
Sweet fruit	0	0	3
Vegetables (without starch)	1	1	1
Starchy vegetables (roots, cauliflower, etc.)	2	1	1
Milk	3	3	3
Dairy products	3	3	3
Cheese	0	3	0
Eggs	0	0	0
Walnuts, hazelnuts, almonds, peanuts	0	0	3

Yogurt	Plant oils	Sugar, sugary foods	Bread, potatoes, rice, noodles	Sour fruit, tomato paste	Sweet fruit	Vegetables (without starch)	Starchy vegetables (roots, cauliflower, etc.)	Milk	Dairy products	Cheese	Eggs	Walnuts, hazelnuts, almonds, peanuts
0	1	0	3	3	0	1	2	3	3	0	0	0
2	1	0	3	3	0	1	1	3	3	3	0	0
0	0	0	2	3	3	1	1	3	3	0	0	3
	3	3	2	2	3	1	1	0	0	0	0	0
3		3	1	2	3	1	1	0	0	0	2	1
3	3		3	3	3	2	3	3	3	3	0	3
2	1	3		3	3	1	1	3	3	2	3	3
2	2	3	3		3	2	3	0	3	3	0	3
3	3	3	3	3		2	3	3	3	3	0	3
1	1	2	1	2	2		1	3	2	1	1	1
1	1	3	1	3	3	1		2	2	2	3	1
0	0	3	3	0	3	3	2		0	0	0	0
0	0	3	3	3	3	2	2	0		1	3	3
0	0	3	2	3	3	1	2	0	1		0	3
0	2	0	3	0	0	1	3	0	3	0		0
0	1	3	3	3	3	1	1	0	3	3	0	

Cleansing Tea for a 3-Week Treatment

- 2 big glasses water
- 1 bunch parsley
- 1 handful artichoke leaves, fresh or dried
- 1 bunch cornsilk
- 1 handful cherry stems
- 4 avocado leaves

Boil the water, then add all ingredients and boil for another 2 minutes.

Use:

Week 1: One cup 1–2 hours before bedtime and one cup when you get up in the morning. Drink the tea on four days during the first week (every other day).

Week 2: One cup 1–2 hours before bedtime and one when you get up in the morning. Drink the tea on three days during the second week (a 2-day interval).

Week 3: One cup 1–2 hours before bedtime and one when you get up in the morning. Drink the tea only one day during the third week.

Note: *During this treatment, you should not eat any animal products. Also avoid carbohydrates, or consume only small amounts. Instead, I recommend drinking about 1–2 quarts of water a day and eating plenty of vegetables. Breathe in and out deeply, and do relaxation and stretching exercises a few times a day. Avoid strenuous physical activity.*

Testimonials from People Who Have Taken Part in the Beauty and Face Yoga Program

"It all starts with proper deep breathing. Once you learn how to slow down, you will see how quickly you change. You'll notice that your back is straighter, you're not as tired, and it is easier to feel happy. I'm confident that you'll find valuable information in Lourdes Doplito Çabuk's book that you can work into your everyday life. Slowing down is one of those things. I can't claim that it was easy for me. But when I breathe in and manage to think about 'nothing,' and do the Baby Pose at the same time, everything is much simpler. You'll notice the change when you start to slow down, and beauty and everything else will follow!"

— *Tuluhan Tekelioglu, journalist*

"I have to admit that despite my best intentions to accept it, I have had trouble coming to terms with my sinking eyebrows and the wrinkles around my lips and on my neck, especially since my thirty-fifth birthday. Still, I can't understand women my age who go under the knife or have Botox treatments, and eventually mutate into assembly-line androids. Lourdes came into my life when I started thinking about healthier and more natural methods. I met her during one of her seminars. As she talked about natural ways to maintain health and beauty, the participants hung on her every word, enthralled.

What she was talking about was a great concept, and at the same time very simple. Lourdes herself is the perfect illustration of her program, especially when you think about her age and her six grandchildren. During that seminar, I decided I needed to take one of her classes.

In the class, we learned not just how to exercise our facial muscles, but also how to become more vital from the inside out, and how to defy the passage of time. The abdominal, spinal, and breathing exercises changed my complexion and my body tissue. It would be wrong to think this was easy, or some kind of miracle. But I've been doing the exercises regularly since the end of the course, and the results are outstanding. When I look at pictures of myself from 2 years ago, I can see a 70 percent improvement. That's the reward for my persistence."

— *Esra Koyuncu, feng shui expert*

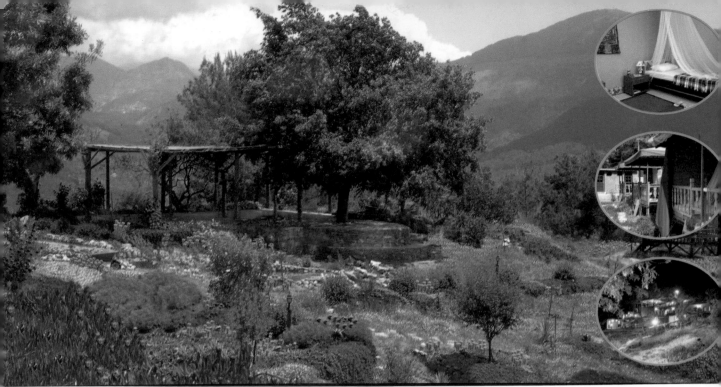

Alanya, Siddashram Yoga C⬤

Lourdes Julian Doplito Çabuk
teaches yoga purification and detoxification in Alanya
at the Siddashram yoga center, and Beauty and Face Yoga at the
Siddashram yoga center in Istanbul (Nişantaşi), Turkey.

Tel: +(90) 212-230-1547   +(90) 533-682-0174
GSM: +(90) 533-777-8640
Website: www.siddashramyogacenter.com
email: info@siddashramyogacenter.com
beautyyoga2000@yahoo.com
lourdescabuk@gmail.com
31901050617358